Acupressure for Women

Womens Wellness Publishing, LLC
www.womenswellnesspublishing.com
www.facebook.com/wwpublishing

Mention of specific companies or products in this book does not suggest endorsement by the author or publisher. Internet addresses and telephone numbers for resources provided in this book were accurate at the time it went to press.

Cover design by Rebecca Rose

ISBN 978-1-939013-80-4

Note: The information in this book is meant to complement the advice and guidance of your physician, not replace it. It is very important that women who have medical problems be evaluated by a physician. If you are under the care of a physician, you should discuss any major changes in your regimen with him or her. Because this is a book and not a medical consultation, keep in mind that the information presented here may not apply in your particular case. In view of individual medical requirements, new research, and government regulations, it is the responsibility of the reader to validate health practices and treatments with a physician or health service.

D1548771

Acknowledgements

I want to give a huge thanks to my amazing editors Kendra Chun and Sandra K. Friend for their incredibly helpful assistance with putting this book together. I also greatly appreciate my fantastic Creative Director, Rebecca Richards, as well as Letitia Truslow, my wonderful Director of Media Relations. I enjoyed working with all of them and found their help indispensable in creating this exceptional book for women. Most of all, I want to thank God and Jesus Christ for their love and blessings.

Table of Contents

Part I:
What is Acupressure?

1

Understanding Acupressure and How It Benefits Women's Health

The ancient Chinese art of acupuncture originated over 5,000 years ago. Its tremendous therapeutic benefits have been proven over thousands of years. More recently, many scientific research studies have validated the effectiveness of this treatment for more than a hundred conditions ranging from hormonal imbalances and menopause-related problems such as insomnia, depression, and anxiety to hair loss, food cravings, and even easing the side effects of cancer-related chemotherapy.

Many of my patients who wanted to combine Eastern and Western healing theories have benefited greatly from this approach. I have utilized many nutritional therapies, sometimes including Chinese herbal products and formulas, as well as Western-based ones, to help bring my patients back into hormonal balance.

A number of my patients have also benefited from acupuncture and acupressure. Not only do these treatments help to reduce menopause-related symptoms, PMS, menstrual cramps, and other female hormonal issues without causing any of the negative side effects associated with conventional HRT, but they can be used in conjunction with any other treatments a woman may also be utilizing.

The traditional Chinese medicine model maintains that everything in your body is governed by two equally important, but opposing, principles — **yin** and **yang**.

Yin is associated with the feminine. It regulates the fluids, blood, and tissues of your body, as well as its structural components, such as flesh, tendons, and bones. It is also is associated with coolness, moisture, quiet, calm, and receptivity.

Conversely, yang is associated with masculinity. It regulates your body's energy, and is associated with heat, dryness, and assertiveness.

Balance between yin and yang is essential if you are to achieve and maintain optimal health and wellbeing. In young, healthy women, the balance between these two polar opposites is maintained almost effortlessly, because these women are usually energetically healthy. Because they have such great reserves of yin and yang during youth, they can maintain a state of being either very yin or very yang in response to the stresses and demands of their lives for several years. For example, they can engage in intense, yang-like activities, such as studying hard, working overtime, or long, strenuous periods of exercise, without depleting their yin. However, too many long hours and over-doing it will begin to accumulate and eventually manifest symptomatically.

As you begin to reach the menopause transition and menopause itself, it becomes increasingly difficult to maintain an optimal yin-yang balance. During this time, it is common to lose this balance and go to either end of the spectrum. You may experience yin deficiency and adequate yang or abundant yin with very little yang.

Many women with yin deficiency will begin to experience symptoms as estrogen levels (a yin-like element) begin to decline. As a result, their body starts to feel much more yang. This can show up as hot flashes, night sweats, vaginal and tissue dryness, insomnia, mood swings, and tighter, tenser muscles, as well as thinning of skin, hair, bones, and connective tissue, resulting in painful and achy joints. In fact, women who are extremely yin deficient may find that even the slightest energy imbalances can result in an increased risk of disease and illness.

In contrast, women with abundant yin reserves who start to have a deficiency of yang properties will start to retain fluid and gain weight more readily. While they have a more peaceful and calm temperament, they may lack libido, vitality, joie de vivre, and even mental acuity. In Western medicine, we describe this difference with a chemical and physiological model, while in traditional Chinese medicine; it is described in terms of an energetic imbalance.

Estrogen is such a powerful substance that I have come to think of it as practically synonymous with yin, energetically speaking. Women who have estrogen dominance during the premenopause also face a difficult challenge, as they are combating symptoms of estrogen excess, which can escalate out-of-control as the condition becomes more and more extreme. Fortunately, acupuncture, and its sister healing technique, acupressure, can help to restore the yin-yang balance.

Chi: The Rivers of Life

Acupuncture is based on the belief that your health is predicated by a balance of **chi** (life energy) flowing throughout your body. It is different yet similar to electromagnetic energy. Health occurs when the chi is equally distributed throughout the body and is present in sufficient amounts. Chi is thought to energize all the cells and tissues of the body.

Both yin and yang energy (or chi) circulate through your body along 12 major pathways called **meridians**. This distribution system is analogous to blood and lymph vessels except that the latter distribute fluid and the meridians distribute chi which is a subtle energy. Thus, meridians move energy through the body like invisible rivers. They flow deep into the interior of the body through the organ systems and, at times, surface on the skin. The place where the energy surfaces on the skin is called the **acupuncture point**. The electrical resistance of the skin at these points is slightly different from that of the surrounding skin.

Disease is thought to occur when the energy flow through a meridian stops or is blocked. The corresponding internal organ system manifests symptoms of disease. The meridian flow can be corrected by stimulating the points on the surface of the skin. These points can be treated either by hand massage, insertion of needles or electrical stimulus. When the normal flow of energy through the body is resumed, the body is believed to heal itself spontaneously.

The Meridian System

The major meridians are the kidney, bladder, heart, small intestine, large intestine, spleen/pancreas, stomach, lung, liver, gall bladder, pericardium (blood vessels), and triple warmer (san jiao). Of these, the kidney, spleen/ pancreas, and liver meridians are key for women in any phase of the hormonal cycle, be it menstruation or menopause.

In traditional Chinese medicine, the **kidneys** are seen as the foundation of the strength and energy of the body. The reserve energy of the body is also contained within the kidneys. As such, the kidneys regulate the sexual organs (ovaries) and their reproductive function. Healthy menstruation, healthy reproduction, and an easy menopause are all dependent on healthy kidney function. The other source of female hormones—the adrenal glands—are also part of the kidney function.

Given their preeminent role as the root source of your body's energy, the kidneys are the foundation of all yin and yang qualities. Similarly to what I described earlier in this chapter, when **kidney yin** is sufficient, it has a heat-reducing, calming, cooling, moisturizing, and tissue-building effect on your body. When kidney yin is deficient, the tissues of the body are overheated, drier, and more congested. This leads to hot flashes, night sweats, insomnia, and vaginal dryness. The emotions of a menopausal woman suffering from kidney yin deficiency tend toward nervousness, anxiety, irritation, and fear.

When **kidney yang** is deficient, menopausal women suffer from low libido, urinary incontinence, loss of mental acuity, low back pain, and pale complexion. This indicates that the warming and energizing yang function of the kidneys is out of balance.

The **spleen/pancreas meridian** supplies the kidney yang by supporting healthy digestion and absorption of nutrients. If your digestive function is weak, you are more likely to lack in kidney yang. You are also likely to have low willpower and be indecisive. If you are still in your active, reproductive years, you may experience menstrual problems, including irregular and heavy periods, due to weak spleen/pancreas energy.

Liver meridian imbalances can also contribute to menstrual, pre- and perimenopausal, and menopausal symptoms. An overheated, congested, or inflamed liver, overtaxed by an unhealthy diet, alcohol, drugs, or toxins, can put additional stress on the kidneys. The kidneys must produce extra yin fluids to act as a coolant or decongestant to the liver. Over time, this drains your body's yin, depleting your kidney's supply of reserve energy. This, in turn, greatly aggravates menopausal symptoms.

Treating Meridian Points with Acupuncture or Acupressure

Along all the meridians, there are places where the energy surfaces on the skin. These are called acupuncture points. Stimulating these points on the surface of the skin with a fine needle (acupuncture), laser colored light device, electroacupuncture, or by hand pressure (acupressure) can correct the meridian flow and bring your chi back into balance.

Acupressure is closely related to acupuncture. Both are used to restore the proper flow of chi. Unlike acupuncture, which requires needles and can only be done by a trained practitioner, acupressure uses the application of gentle finger pressure to specific points on the skin. And you can do it yourself!

2

Medical Research Validates the Benefits of Acupuncture

Acupuncture is the most widely studied alternative medicine treatment other than nutritional supplementation. When it comes to stimulating healthy hormone production, restoring proper yin-yang balance with acupuncture or acupressure is a great complement to any supplementation program. It has been found to help a whole host of illnesses and health conditions, ranging from bone health and mood disorders to hot flashes and menstrual cramps.

Let's take a look at the research that exists specifically for treatment from estrogen dominance and estrogen deficiency related conditions.

Acupuncture for Estrogen Dominance

Acupuncture and acupressure have been shown to be highly effective treatment modalities for women suffering from estrogen dominance related issues. These therapies are particularly effective for treating PMS symptoms such as sore and painful breasts, nausea, headaches, menstrual cramps, and anxiety. Acupuncture has also been found to be considerably successful in helping women with hormone-related fertility issues to conceive.

According to a study from the *Archives of Gynecology and Obstetrics*, acupuncture was effective in significantly reducing a wide variety of PMS symptoms, including anxiety, gastrointestinal complaints, insomnia, nausea, and premenstrual headaches. In fact, nearly 79 percent of the women receiving acupuncture enjoyed relief, as compared to less than six percent in the control group.

A study from the *Journal of Advanced Nursing* found that acupressure was also helpful in alleviating PMS symptoms, namely menstrual cramps and anxiety. Researchers divided 69 girls into two groups. The first group received 20 minutes of acupressure on a spot three finger-widths above the ankle bone on the inside of the leg. The second group was given 20 minutes of bed rest. For the next four to six week, the participants were asked perform the acupressure on themselves or to rest, depending on which group they were in. At the end of the study period, 87 percent of the participants found the acupressure helpful in reducing pain associated with PMS.

A similar study from the *Journal of Traditional Chinese Medicine* also found that acupressure was highly effective for reducing pain associated with menstrual cramps. Researchers divided 216 teenage girls aged 14 to 18 years into three groups. One group received acupressure, the other received ibuprofen, and the third received "false" acupressure. Both the acupressure group and the ibuprofen group enjoyed a 72 percent decrease in menstrual pain, as compared to the "false" group, who saw a 58 percent reduction in pain.

Another medical study using acupuncture for the treatment of menstrual cramps and pain was done by Dr. Joseph Helms, a family practitioner in Berkeley, California. In his study, 43 women were divided into four groups. All these women were using medication to control menstrual pain. One group of women received treatment with the acupuncture points necessary to control the menstrual pain symptoms. The other three groups received either false acupuncture treatment or no treatment.

At the end of this 12-month study, 90 percent of those receiving real acupuncture treatment reported rapid and significant symptom relief. This included relief of cramping, nausea, back pain, headaches, and fluid retention. In contrast, only 36 percent of the women who received the false acupuncture treatments said that they noted symptom relief.

Other physicians using acupuncture and acupressure to treat fibroids symptoms note similar results. Good results are more likely to occur in women with mild to moderate symptoms. Acupressure may not be as effective in women with more severe and advanced cases; these women may need to use Western medical treatments along with a variety of self-help therapies.

Finally, acupuncture is widely accepted for its ability to support fertility treatments. One such study published in *Fertility and Sterility* found that of the 80 patients undergoing in-vitro fertilization (IVF) who also received acupuncture for six weeks, 42 percent became pregnant, as compared to just 26 percent of those women who did not receive acupuncture.

Acupuncture for Estrogen Deficiency/Yin Deficiency

There is a plethora of research studies on acupuncture and acupressure use to treat a myriad of menopause-related conditions, especially hot flashes and insomnia.

In one study from China, 300 women aged 41 to 60 were treated for hot flashes and other menopause-related symptoms. According to the survey, after three 20 minute acupuncture sessions, 51 percent of the women were cured, 28 percent had marked improvement, 18 percent were improved, and just 3 percent of the women felt the treatment was ineffective.

Another study from Sweden found that the frequency of hot flashes decreased by 50 percent in 24 women who had been treated with electro-stimulation or needle-insertion acupuncture. After three months, the women treated with electrostimulation still enjoyed a reduction in their hot flashes, while those treated with needles had a slight rebound in their symptoms. Similarly, a pilot study conducted at the University Hospital of Geneva in Switzerland reported that acupuncture treatments that had been given to 11 women for relief from menopausal symptoms lasted up to three months.

A growing body of clinical evidence also shows that acupressure is effective in treating insomnia and sleep-related issues. A study published in *Neurophysiologie Clinique* reported that stimulus of a specific acupressure point on the wrist resulted in decreased wakefulness and increased total sleep time. A similar study published in the *Journal of Chinese Medicine* reported that 13 night-crying infants all ceased night crying after only three treatment sessions.

Ease Effects of Chemotherapy

Acupuncture, particularly electroacupuncture, has been shown to help prevent and treat nausea and vomiting associated with chemotherapy. According to a study from the *Journal of Alternative and Complementary Medicine*, 27 cancer patients who experienced severe and refractory nausea and vomiting from chemotherapy were given electroacupuncture at their next chemotherapy treatment. More than 96 percent of the patients had significantly less nausea and vomiting, and more than a third of the patients (37 percent) reported no vomiting at all.

3

How to Perform Acupressure

All of the acupressure exercises in this book can be done by you or by a friend following the simple instructions in this section. It is safe, painless, and does not require the use of needles. It can be used without the years of specialized training needed for insertion of needles.

Acupressure should be done when you are relaxed. Your room should be warm and quiet. Make sure your hands are clean and nails trimmed (to avoid bruising). If your hands are cold, rinse them under warm water.

Work on the side of the body that has the most discomfort. If both sides are equally uncomfortable, choose either side. Just working on one side will relieve the symptoms on both sides. Energy or information seems to transfer from one side to the other.

Look carefully at the illustration for the exercise. When you locate the correct point you are treating, press the point firmly with the tips of both your index and middle fingers. Hold the point for one to three minutes. If you feel any resistance or tension in the area, increase the pressure slightly. If your hands start to tense up or become tired, reduce the pressure a little bit. The acupressure point may feel tender; this means the energy pathway or meridian is blocked.

During the treatment, the tenderness in the point should slowly fade. You may also have a sense of energy radiating from this point into the body. Many women describe this sensation as very pleasant. Do not worry if you don't feel it, not everyone does. The main goal is some relief from your symptoms. Breathe gently while doing each exercise. The point that you are to hold is shown in the drawing accompanying the exercise. All of these points correspond to specific points on the acupressure meridians. You may apply acupressure to the points once a day, or more if you continue to have symptoms.

Part II:
Acupressure Exercises for Specific Conditions

4

Balances the Entire Reproductive System

Exercise 1: Balances the Entire Reproductive System

This exercise alleviates all menstrual complaints, balances the energy of the female reproductive tract, and relieves low back pain and abdominal discomfort.

Equipment: This exercise uses a knotted hand towel to put pressure on hard to reach areas of the back. Place the knotted towel on these points while your two hands are on other points. This increases your ability to unblock the energy pathways of your body.

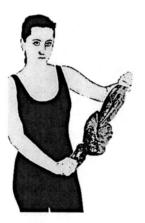
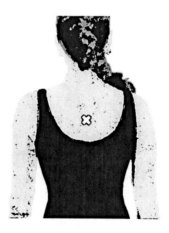

Lie on the floor with your knees up. As you lie down, place the towel between the shoulder blades on your spine. Hold each step 1 to 3 minutes.

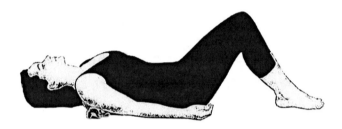

Cross your arms on your chest. Press your thumbs against the right and left inside upper arms.

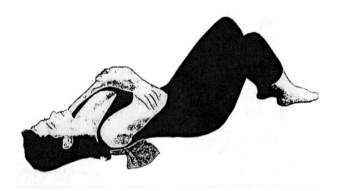

Left hand holds point at the base of the sternum (breastbone).

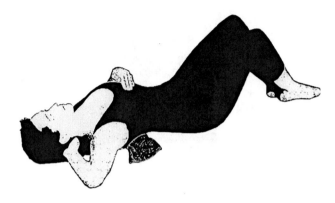

Right hand holds point at the base of the head (at the junction of the spine and the skull).

Interlace your fingers. Place them below your breasts. Fingertips should press directly against the body.

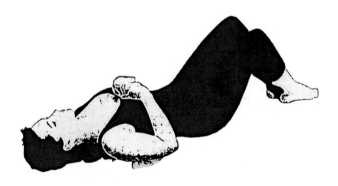

Move the knotted towel along the spine to the waistline.

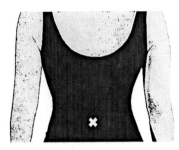

Left hand should be placed at the top of the pubic bone, pressing down.

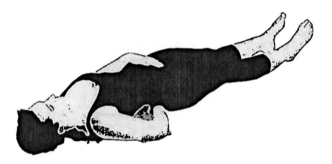

Right hand holds point on tailbone.

Exercise 2: Balances the energy of the reproductive organs

This exercise balances the energy of the reproductive organs. This exercise also relieves menstrual cramps and low back pain by balancing points on the bladder meridian.

Sit on the floor and prop your back against a wall or a heavy piece of furniture. Hold each step for 1 to 3 minutes.

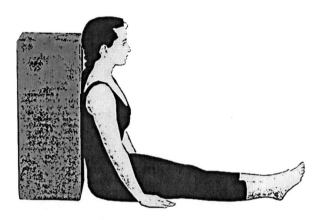

Alternative method: Lie on the floor and put your lower legs over the seat of a chair. Follow the exercise from that position.

Place left hand 1 inch above the waist on the muscle to the left side of the spine (muscle will feel firm and ropelike). Place right hand behind crease of the left knee.

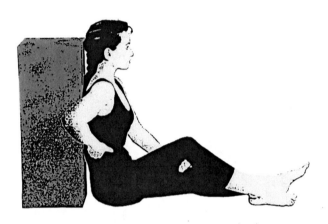

Left hand stays in the same position. Right hand is placed on the center of the back of the left calf. This is just below the fullest part of the calf.

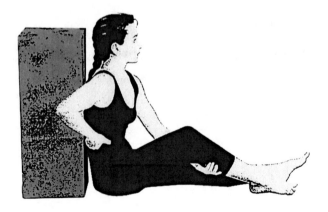

Left hand remains 1 inch above the waist on the muscle to the side of the spine. Right hand is placed just below the ankle bone on the outside of the left heel.

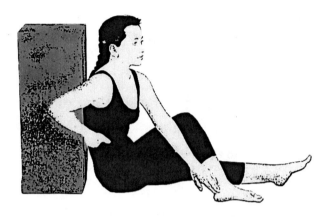

Left hand remains 1 inch above the waist on the muscle to the side of the spine. Right hand holds the front and back of the left little toe at the nail.

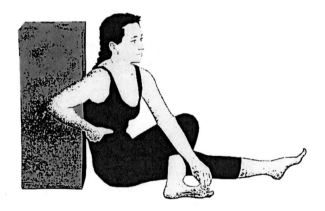

5

PMS (Premenstrual Syndrome)

Exercise 1: Relieves PMS Related Cramps, Bloating, Fluid Retention, and Weight Gain

This sequence of points balances the energy flow of the spleen meridian. It relieves bloating and fluid retention and helps to minimize weight gain in the premenstrual period. It is also effective for relieving menstrual cramps.

Sit up and prop your back against a chair, or lie down and put your lower legs on a chair. Hold each step for 1 to 3 minutes

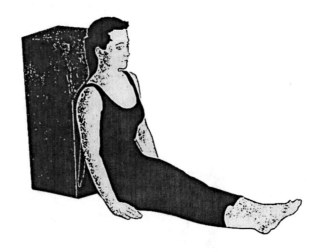

Left hand is placed in the crease of the groin where you bend your leg, one-third to one-half way between the hip bone and the outside edge of the pubic bone. Right hand holds a spot 2 to 3 inches above the knee.

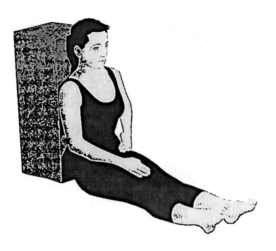

Left hand remains in the crease of the groin. Right hand holds point below inner part of knee. To find the point, follow the curve of the bone just below the knee. Hold the underside of the curve with your fingers.

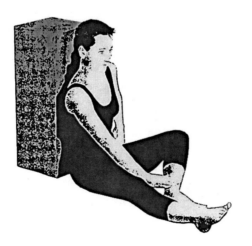

Left hand remains in the crease of the groin. Right hand holds the inside of the shin. To find this point, go four finger widths above the ankle bone. The point is just above the top finger.

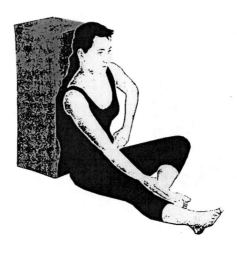

Left hand remains in the crease of the groin. Right hand holds the edge of the instep. To find the point, follow the big toe bone up until you hit a knobby, prominent small bone.

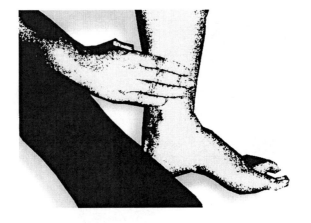

Left hand remains in the crease of the groin.

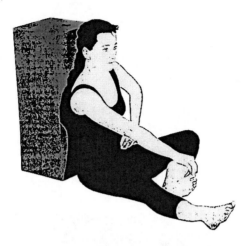

Right hand holds the big toe over the nail, front and back of the toe.

Exercise 2: Relieves Premenstrual Nausea

This exercise relieves premenstrual nausea. This usually occurs in conjunction with cramps and low back pain.

Lie on the floor or sit up. Left index finger is placed in navel and pointed slightly toward the head.

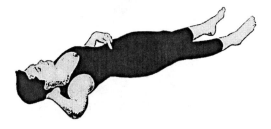

Right hand holds point at the base of the head. Hold these points 1 to 3 minutes.

Exercise 3: Relieves PMS Related Acne

This exercise relieves PMS related acne and helps to relieve hives.

Sit on the floor with the knees bent. Hold each step 1 to 3 minutes. Left hand holds left calf. Right hand holds right calf.

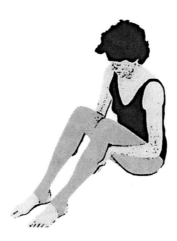

Cross arms. Left hand holds right calf. Right hand holds left calf.

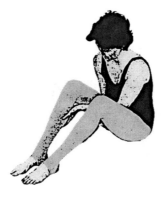

Exercise 4: Relieves PMS Related Depression, Headaches, Tightness of Neck and Shoulders, and Hypoglycemia

The neck and shoulders generally carry a great deal of tension. Tightness in this area can act as a bottleneck and impede the energy flow of the entire body. Thus the entire body is energized by this exercise. It also relieves depression.

A major treatment point for hypoglycemia is worked on in this exercise. This may held reduce the excessive cravings for sweets that some women notice before their periods.

Sit comfortably or lie down. Hold each step 1 to 3 minutes. Left hand holds point at the top of the shoulder blade, 1 to 2 inches to the side of the spine. The point is between the shoulder blade and the spine. It may feel firm and resistant. Right hand holds the same point on the right side.

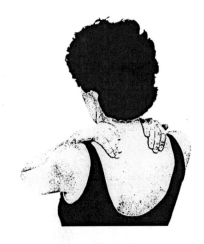

Left hand holds points slightly to the back of the top of the shoulder where the neck meets the shoulder. Right hand holds the same point on the right side.

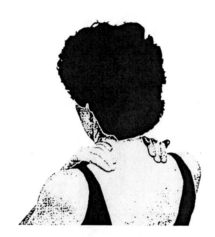

Left hand holds the point halfway up the neck, fingers sit on the muscle next to the spine. Right hand holds the same point on the right side.

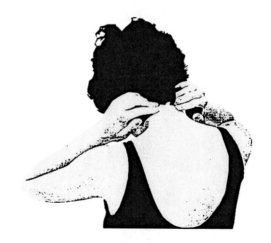

Left hand holds the point at the base of the skull 1 to 2 inches out from the spine. Right hand holds the same point on the right side.

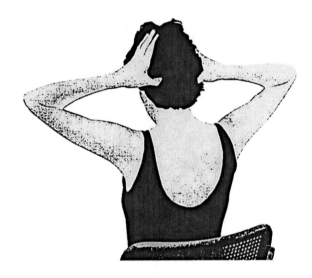

6

Menstrual Cramps

Exercise 1: Relieves Cramps, Bloating, Fluid Retention, Weight Gain

This sequence of points balances the points on the spleen meridian. It helps to relieve menstrual cramps. It also relieves bloating and fluid retention and helps to minimize weight gain in the period leading up to menstruation.

Sit up and prop your back against a chair, or lie down and put your lower legs on a chair. Hold each step for 1 to 3 minutes

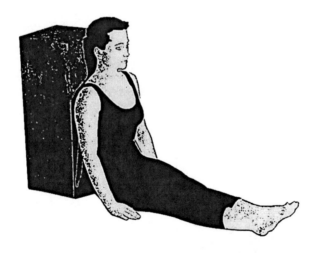

Left hand is placed in the crease of the groin where you bend your leg, one-third to one-half way between the hip bone and the outside edge of the pubic bone. Right hand holds a spot 2 to 3 inches above the knee.

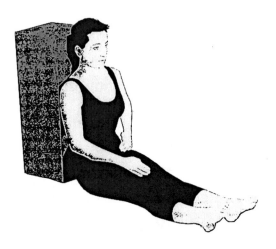

Left hand remains in the crease of the groin. Right hand holds point below inner part of knee. To find the point, follow the curve of the bone just below the knee. Hold the underside of the curve with your fingers.

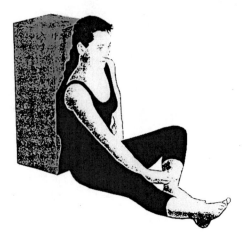

Left hand remains in the crease of the groin. Right hand holds the inside of the shin. To find this point, go four finger widths above the ankle bone. The point is just above the top finger.

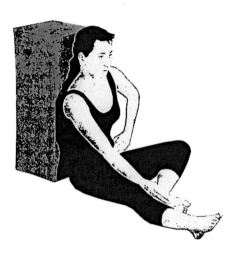

Left hand remains in the crease of the groin. Right hand holds the edge of the instep. To find the point, follow the big toe bone up until you hit a knobby, prominent small bone.

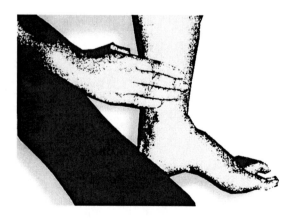

Left hand remains in the crease of the groin.

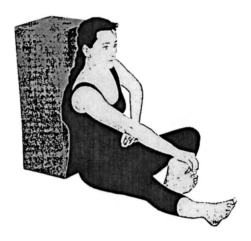

Right hand holds the big toe over the nail, front and back of the toe.

Exercise 2: Relieves Nausea

This exercise relieves the nausea and digestive symptoms that often occur with menstrual cramps and low back pain.

Lie on the floor or sit up. Hold these points 1 to 3 minutes.

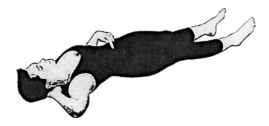

Left index finger is placed in navel and pointed slightly toward the head. Right hand holds point at the base of the head.

Exercise 3: Relieves Menstrual Fatigue

This sequence of points relieves the **fatigue** that women experience just prior to the onset of their menstrual period. Tiredness may last through the first few days of menstruation for many women. This exercise can also help to relieve menstrual anxiety and depression. Caution: The second step in this sequence has traditionally been forbidden for use by pregnant women after their first trimester.

Sit up and prop your back against a chair. Hold each step for 1 to 3 minutes.

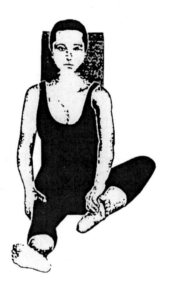

Left hand holds point at the base of the ball of the right foot. This point is located between the two pads of the foot.

Left hand holds the point midway between the inside of the right anklebone and the Achilles tendon. The Achilles tendon is located at the back of the ankle.

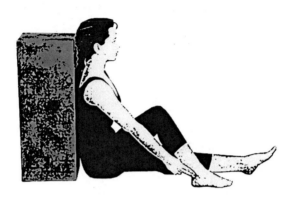

Left hand holds point below right knee. This point is located four finger-widths below the kneecap toward the outside of the shinbone. It is sensitive to the touch in many people.

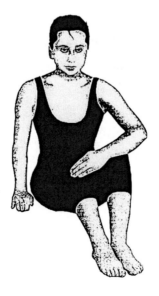

Exercise 4: Relieves Low Back Pain and Menstrual Cramps

This exercise relieves menstrual cramps and low back pain by balancing points on the bladder meridian. It also balances the energy of the female reproductive tract.

Sit on the floor and prop your back against a wall or a heavy piece of furniture. Hold each step for 1 to 3 minutes.

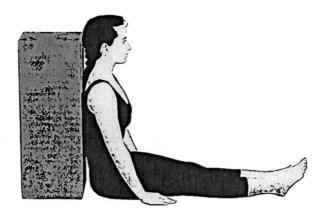

Alternative method: Lie on the floor and put your lower legs over the seat of a chair. Follow the exercise from that position.

Place left hand 1 inch above the waist on the muscle to the left side of the spine (muscle will feel firm and ropelike). Place right hand behind crease of the left knee.

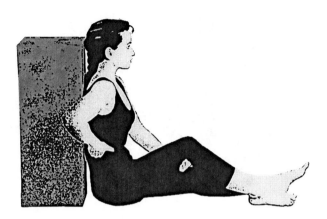

Left hand stays in the same position. Right hand is placed on the center of the back of the left calf. This is just below the fullest part of the calf.

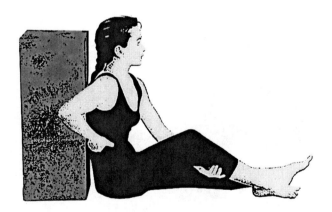

Left hand remains 1 inch above the waist on the muscle to the side of the spine. Right hand is placed just below the ankle bone on the outside of the left heel.

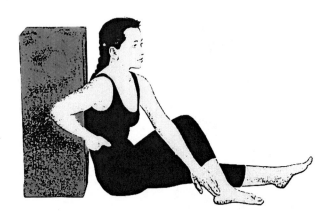

Left hand remains 1 inch above the waist on the muscle to the side of the spine. Right hand holds the front and back of the left little toe at the nail.

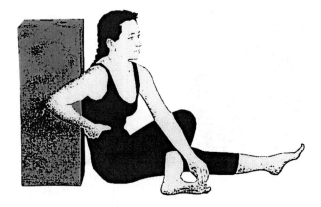

7

Heavy and Irregular Menstruation

Exercise 1: Relieves Excessive Menstrual Bleeding

This exercise has been used traditionally in controlling excessive uterine bleeding.

Sit upright on a chair. Hold each step for 1 to 3 minutes. Bend over at the waist with left hand holding point in front of ankle bone. Move hand slowly along points on leg.

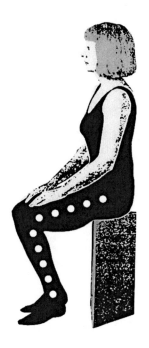
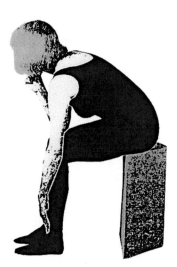

Move left hand slowly on points to the top of the thigh. Repeat on the right side with right hand.

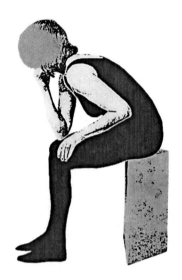 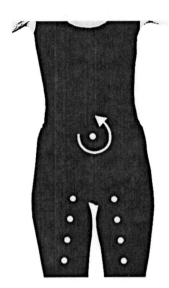

Right hand in middle of thigh points up to groin. Repeat on other side with left hand. Circle area around navel in counterclockwise direction.

Exercise 2: Relieves Thyroid Imbalance

This exercise energizes the thyroid, which can cause excessive menstrual bleeding.

Sit upright on a chair. Hold each step for 1 to 3 minutes. Wrap hands around shoulders with thumbs pressing gently into both sides on top of collarbone.

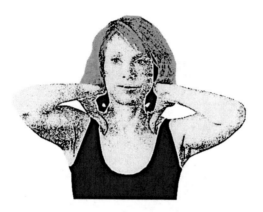

Fingers are in back and press against upper shoulders and shoulder blade area.

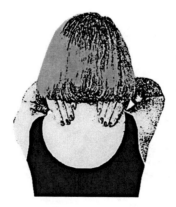

Exercise 3: Use for Relief of Anemia due to Heavy and Irregular Menstruation

This sequence of points is helpful for the treatment of anemia. It involves the stimulation of points on the spleen meridian that affect menstrual problems and blood formation.

Sit upright on a chair. Hold each step for 1 to 3 minutes. Right hand holds point four finger-widths above the ankle bone.

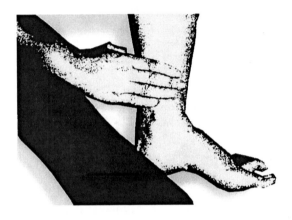

Right hand holds point above and below the nail of the big toe.

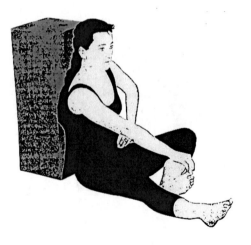

Exercise 4: Relieves Excessive Menstrual Bleeding

This exercise normalizes the energy of reproductive organs by balancing points on the bladder meridian. It also relieves lower back pain and can help to relieve excessive menstrual bleeding.

Sit on the floor and prop your back against a wall or a heavy piece of furniture. Hold each step for 1 to 3 minutes.

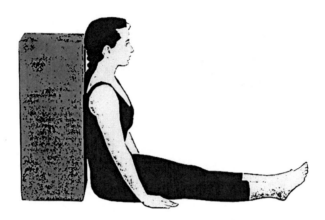

Alternative method: Lie on the floor and put your lower legs over the seat of a chair. Follow the exercise from that position.

Place left hand 1 inch above the waist on the muscle to the left side of the spine (muscle will feel firm and ropelike). Place right hand behind crease of the left knee.

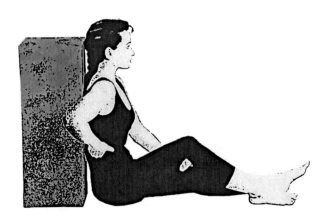

Left hand stays in the same position. Right hand is placed on the center of the back of the left calf. This is just below the fullest part of the calf.

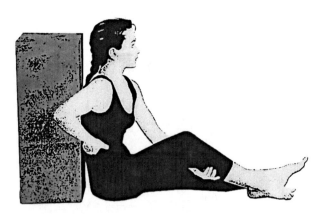

Left hand remains 1 inch above the waist on the muscle to the side of the spine. Right hand is placed just below the ankle bone on the outside of the left heel.

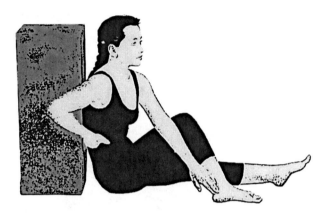

Left hand remains 1 inch above the waist on the muscle to the side of the spine. Right hand holds the front and back of the left little toe at the nail.

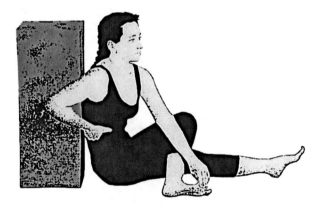

Exercise 5: Use for Relief of Fatigue and Tiredness

This exercise helps to relieve the fatigue and tiredness that commonly accompany heavy menstrual bleeding.

Sit upright on a chair. Hold each step for 1 to 3 minutes. Right hand holds a point directly between the eyebrows, where the bridge of the nose meets the forehead.

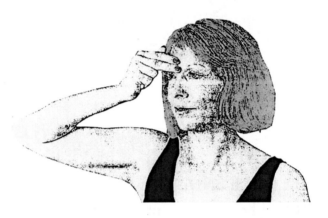

Fingers hold a point below the navel. Measure three finger-widths below the navel to find this point.

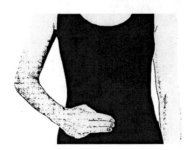

8

Fibroid Tumors

Exercise 1: Relieves pelvic and abdominal discomfort and low back pain seen with fibroid tumors

This exercise is used to balance the energy of the female reproductive tract and relieve all menstrual complaints. It also relieves pelvic and abdominal discomfort and low back pain, which are very common complaints in women with fibroids.

Equipment: This exercise uses a knotted hand towel to put pressure on hard to reach areas of the back. Place the knotted towel on these points while your two hands are on other points. This increases your ability to unblock the energy pathways of your body.

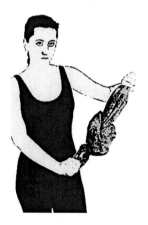 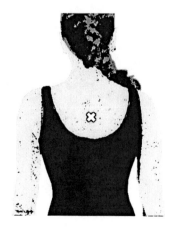

Lie on the floor with your knees up. As you lie down, place the towel between the shoulder blades on your spine. Hold each step 1 to 3 minutes.

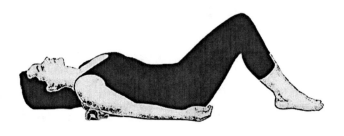

Cross your arms on your chest. Press your thumbs against the right and left inside upper arms.

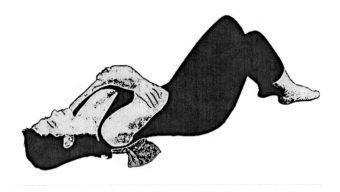

Left hand holds point at the base of the sternum (breastbone).

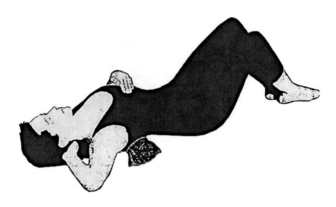

Right hand holds point at the base of the head (at the junction of the spine and the skull).

Interlace your fingers. Place them below your breasts. Fingertips should press directly against the body.

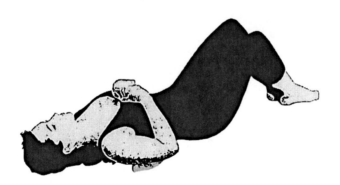

Move the knotted towel along the spine to the waistline.

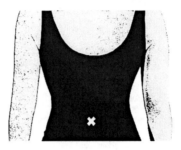

Left hand should be placed at the top of the pubic bone, pressing down.

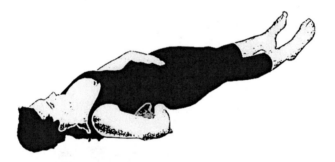

Right hand holds point on tailbone.

Exercise 2: Relieves Pelvic and Abdominal Discomfort and Heavy Menstrual Bleeding seen with Fibroids

This sequence balances points on the spleen meridian, used in acupressure to relieve pelvic and abdominal discomfort associated with fibroids and relieve menstrual cramps. Stimulation of these points also relieves fluid retention, premenstrual bloating and helps minimize weight gain in the period leading up to menstruation. In addition, the spleen meridian helps regulate heavy menstrual bleeding commonly seen with fibroids.

Sit up and prop your back against a chair, or lie down and put your lower legs on a chair. Hold each step for 1 to 3 minutes

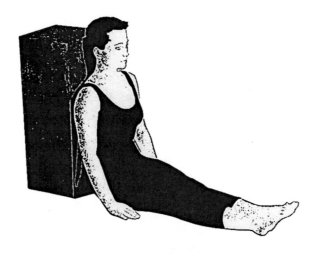

Left hand is placed in the crease of the groin where you bend your leg, one-third to one-half way between the hip bone and the outside edge of the pubic bone. Right hand holds a spot 2 to 3 inches above the knee.

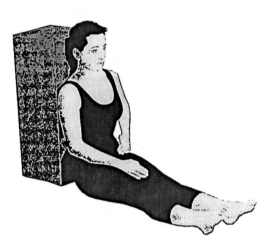

Left hand remains in the crease of the groin. Right hand holds point below inner part of knee. To find the point, follow the curve of the bone just below the knee. Hold the underside of the curve with your fingers.

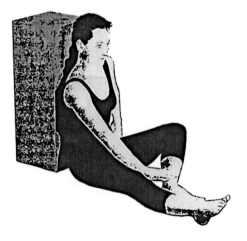

Left hand remains in the crease of the groin. Right hand holds the inside of the shin. To find this point, go four finger widths above the ankle bone. The point is just above the top finger.

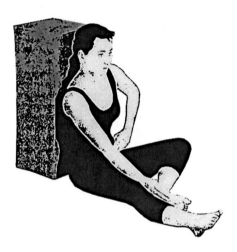

Left hand remains in the crease of the groin. Right hand holds the edge of the instep. To find the point, follow the big toe bone up until you hit a knobby, prominent small bone.

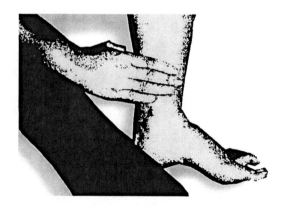

Left hand remains in the crease of the groin.

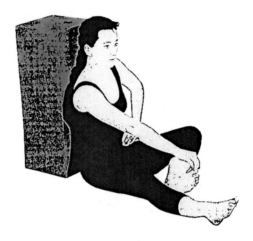

Right hand holds the big toe over the nail, front and back of the toe.

Exercise 3: Relieves Menstrual Fatigue and Stress due to Fibroids

This sequence of points relieves the fatigue that women experience just prior to the onset of the menstrual period. For many women, tiredness may last through the first few days of menstruation. Women with heavy menstrual bleeding due to fibroids may tire easily because of blood loss. This exercise can also relieve menstrual anxiety and depression, helpful to women suffering from significant stress in their lives. The second step in this sequence has traditionally been forbidden for use by pregnant women after their first trimester.

Sit up and prop your back against a chair. Hold each step for 1 to 3 minutes. Left hand holds point at the base of the ball of the right foot. This point is located between the two pads of the foot.

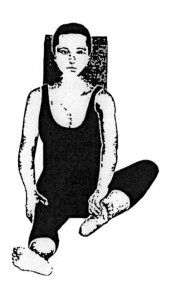

Left hand holds the point midway between the inside of the right anklebone and the Achilles tendon. The Achilles tendon is located at the back of the ankle.

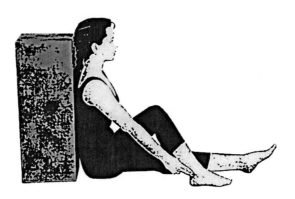

Left hand holds point below right knee. This point is located four finger-widths below the kneecap toward the outside of the shinbone. It is sensitive to the touch in many people.

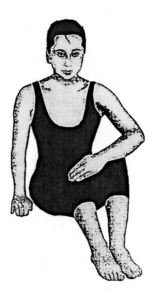

Exercise 4: Relieves Cramps, Digestive Symptoms, and Menstrual Irregularity

This exercise stimulates conception vessel points on the front of the body. These points help relieve constipation, as well as the pain of menstrual cramps caused by fibroids, which can accompany these problems. These points are also used to help treat menstrual irregularity.

Sit or lie in a comfortable position. Place your fingertips on the point two finger-widths below the navel and hold.

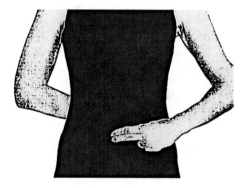

Move your fingertips to the point four finger-widths below the navel and hold.

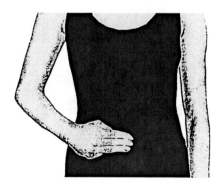

Exercise 5: Relieves Heavy Menstrual Bleeding

This sequence of points is important for the treatment of heavy menstrual flow, which can accompany fibroids. Heavy menstrual bleeding is also a common cause of chronic fatigue and tiredness. This exercise involves the stimulation of points on the spleen meridian, which affect blood formation and menstrual problems.

Sit upright on a chair. Hold each step for 1 to 3 minutes. Right hand holds point four finger-widths above the ankle bone.

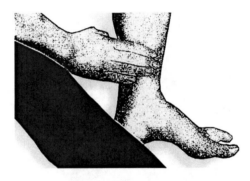

Right hand holds point above and below the nail of the big toe.

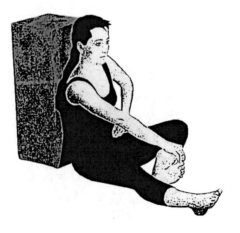

9

Endometriosis

Exercise 1: Relieves the pain of endometriosis

This exercise is used to balance the energy of the female reproductive tract and alleviate all menstrual complaints. It also relieves low back pain and pelvic and abdominal discomfort, which are very common complaints in women with endometriosis.

Equipment: This exercise uses a knotted hand towel to put pressure on hard to reach areas of the back. Place the knotted towel on these points while your two hands are on other points. This increases your ability to unblock the energy pathways of your body.

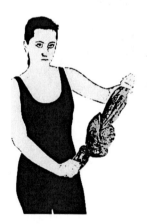 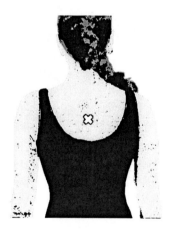

Lie on the floor with your knees up. As you lie down, place the towel between the shoulder blades on your spine. Hold each step 1 to 3 minutes.

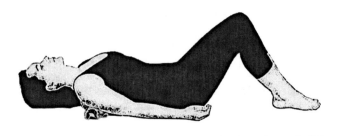

Cross your arms on your chest. Press your thumbs against the right and left inside upper arms.

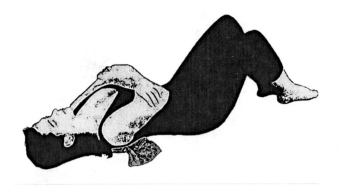

Left hand holds point at the base of the sternum (breastbone).

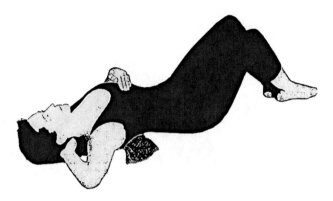

Right hand holds point at the base of the head (at the junction of the spine and the skull).

Interlace your fingers. Place them below your breasts. Fingertips should press directly against the body.

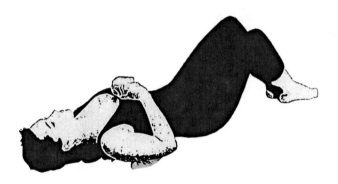

Move the knotted towel along the spine to the waistline.

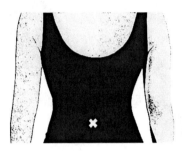

Left hand should be placed at the top of the pubic bone, pressing down.

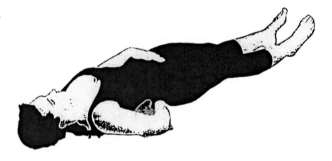

Right hand holds point on tailbone.

Exercise 2: Relieves Cramps, Bloating, Fluid Retention, Weight Gain

This sequence balances the points on the spleen meridian, used in acupressure to relieve menstrual cramps and pelvic and abdominal discomfort associated with endometriosis. Stimulation of these points also relieves premenstrual bloating and fluid retention and helps minimize weight gain in the period leading up to menstruation. The spleen meridian also helps regulate heavy menstrual bleeding.

Sit up and prop your back against a chair, or lie down and put your lower legs on a chair. Hold each step for 1 to 3 minutes

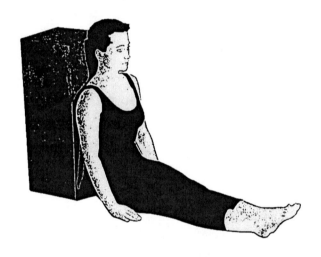

Left hand is placed in the crease of the groin where you bend your leg, one-third to one-half way between the hip bone and the outside edge of the pubic bone. Right hand holds a spot 2 to 3 inches above the knee.

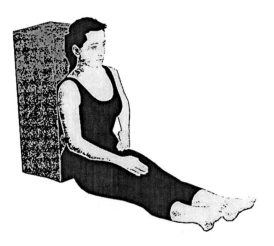

Left hand remains in the crease of the groin. Right hand holds point below inner part of knee. To find the point, follow the curve of the bone just below the knee. Hold the underside of the curve with your fingers.

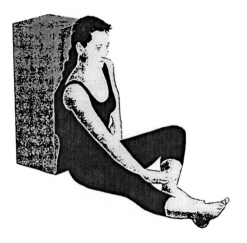

Left hand remains in the crease of the groin. Right hand holds the inside of the shin. To find this point, go four finger widths above the ankle bone. The point is just above the top finger.

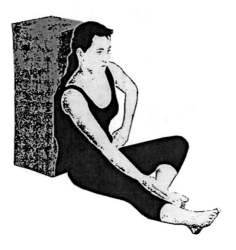

Left hand remains in the crease of the groin. Right hand holds the edge of the instep. To find the point, follow the big toe bone up until you hit a knobby, prominent small bone.

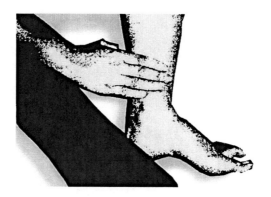

Left hand remains in the crease of the groin.

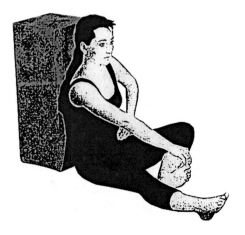

Right hand holds the big toe over the nail, front and back of the toe.

Exercise 3: Relieves Pelvic Tension and Urinary problems of Endometriosis

This exercise relieves menstrual cramps and low back pain by balancing points on the bladder meridian. By balancing the energy of the female reproductive tract the bladder meridian relieves symptoms. These points are also used in Chinese medicine to relieve pelvic tension, and urinary problems, which are often seen with endometriosis.

Sit on the floor and prop your back against a wall or a heavy piece of furniture. Hold each step for 1 to 3 minutes.

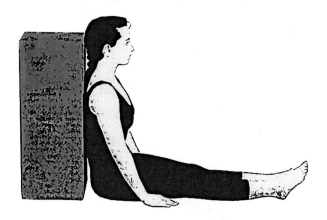

Alternative method: Lie on the floor and put your lower legs over the seat of a chair. Follow the exercise from that position.

Place left hand 1 inch above the waist on the muscle to the left side of the spine (muscle will feel firm and ropelike). Place right hand behind crease of the left knee.

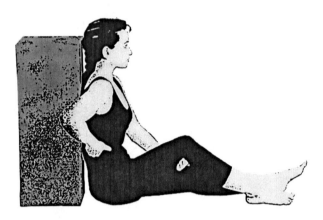

Left hand stays in the same position. Right hand is placed on the center of the back of the left calf. This is just below the fullest part of the calf.

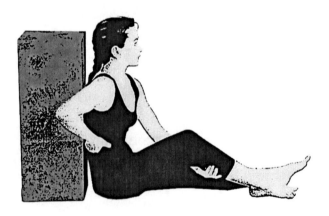

Left hand remains 1 inch above the waist on the muscle to the side of the spine. Right hand is placed just below the ankle bone on the outside of the left heel.

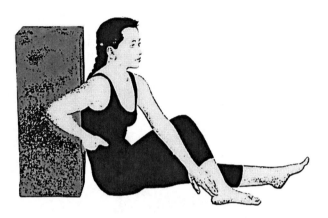

Left hand remains 1 inch above the waist on the muscle to the side of the spine. Right hand holds the front and back of the left little toe at the nail.

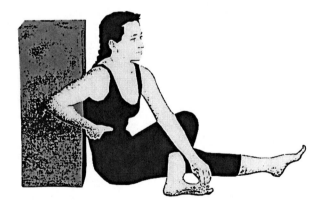

Exercise 4: Relieves Nausea

This exercise relieves the nausea and digestive symptoms that occur when endometriosis invades the small intestines or with cramps and low back pain due to endometriosis.

Lie on the floor or sit up. Hold these points 1 to 3 minutes.

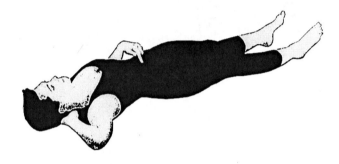

Left index finger is placed in navel and pointed slightly toward the head. Right hand holds point at the base of the head.

Exercise 5: Relieves Menstrual Fatigue and Stress

This sequence of points relieves the fatigue that women experience just prior to the onset of the menstrual period. For many women, tiredness may last through the first few days of menstruation. Women with heavy menstrual bleeding and spotting due to endometriosis may tire easily because of blood loss. This exercise can also relieve menstrual anxiety and depression, helpful to women suffering from significant stress in their lives. Women suffering from endometriosis often complain of excessive stress. The second step in this sequence has traditionally been forbidden for use by pregnant women after their first trimester.

Sit up and prop your back against a chair. Hold each step for 1 to 3 minutes.

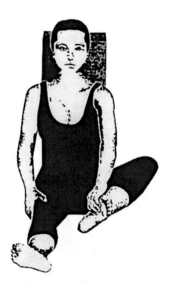

Left hand holds point at the base of the ball of the right foot. This point is located between the two pads of the foot.

Left hand holds the point midway between the inside of the right anklebone and the Achilles tendon. The Achilles tendon is located at the back of the ankle.

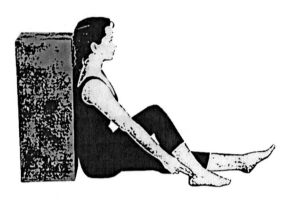

Left hand holds point below right knee. This point is located four finger-widths below the kneecap toward the outside of the shinbone. It is sensitive to the touch in many people.

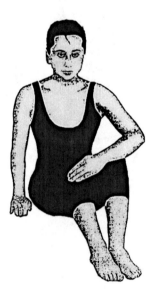

Exercise 6: Relieves Cramps, Digestive Symptoms, and Menstrual Irregularity of endometriosis

This exercise stimulates conception vessel points on the front of the body. These points help relieve the pain of menstrual cramps caused by endometriosis as well as constipation, which can accompany this problems. These points are also used to help treat menstrual irregularity.

Sit or lie in a comfortable position. Place your fingertips on the point two finger-widths below the navel and hold.

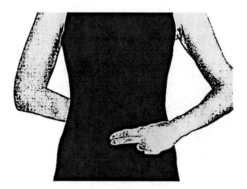

Move your fingertips to the point four finger-widths below the navel and hold.

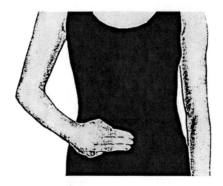

Exercise 7: Relieves Heavy Menstrual Bleeding and spotting due to endometriosis

This sequence of points is important for the treatment of heavy menstrual flow and spotting which can accompany endometriosis. Heavy menstrual bleeding is also a common cause of chronic fatigue and tiredness. This exercise involves the stimulation of points on the spleen meridian, which affect blood formation and menstrual problems.

Sit upright on a chair. Hold each step for 1 to 3 minutes. Right hand holds point four finger-widths above the ankle bone.

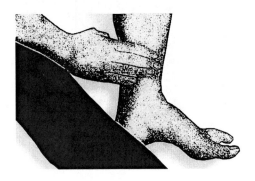

Right hand holds point above and below the nail of the big toe.

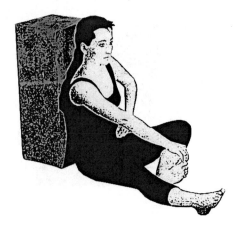

10

Menopause

Exercise 1: Supports Female Health During Menopause

This exercise balances the energy of the female reproductive tract and alleviates all menstrual complaints. It also helps relieve low back pain and abdominal discomfort.

Equipment: This exercise uses a knotted hand towel to put pressure on hard to reach areas of the back. Place the knotted towel on these points while your two hands are on other points. This increases your ability to unblock the energy pathways of your body.

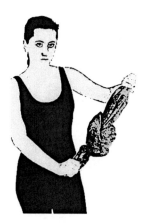
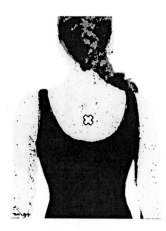

Lie on the floor with your knees up. As you lie down, place the towel between the shoulder blades on your spine. Hold each step 1 to 3 minutes.

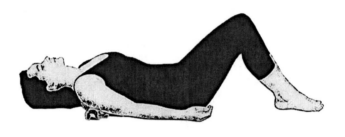

Cross your arms on your chest. Press your thumbs against the right and left inside upper arms.

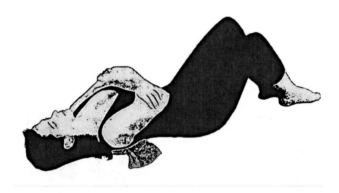

Left hand holds point at the base of the sternum (breastbone).

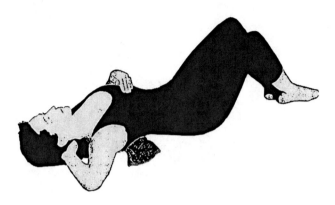

Right hand holds point at the base of the head (at the junction of the spine and the skull).

Interlace your fingers. Place them below your breasts. Fingertips should press directly against the body.

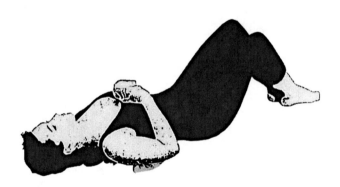

Move the knotted towel along the spine to the waistline.

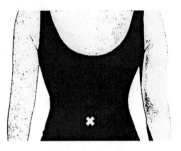

Left hand should be placed at the top of the pubic bone, pressing down.

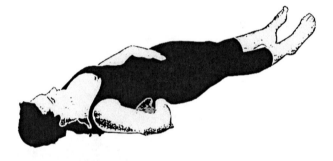

Right hand holds point on tailbone.

Exercise 2: Relieves Hot Flashes and Emotional Tension

This exercise helps relieve hot flashes by stimulating the entire endocrine system. It involves a very powerful point for the pituitary gland, the master regulator of the ovaries. This point also helps relax the emotional tension that many women feel during early menopause and relieves eye strain, headaches, and hay fever.

Sit upright on a chair. Right hand holds point directly between the eyebrows, where the bridge of the nose meets the forehead. Hold the point for 1 to 3 minutes

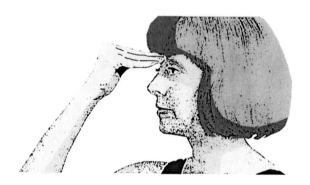

Exercise 3: Relieves Hot Flashes, Menopausal Fatigue, Anxiety, and Depression

This exercise helps relieve hot flashes as well as menopause related fatigue, insomnia, anxiety, and depression. The exercise will also relieve fatigue, anxiety, and depression women may experience prior to their menstrual periods.

Right hand holds point in the center of your breast bone, at the level of the heart. Your fingers will fit into the indentations in this bone.
Sit up and prop your back against a chair. Hold each step 1 to 3 minutes.

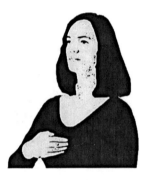

Right hand holds point at the base of the ball of the right foot. This point is located between the two pads of the foot.

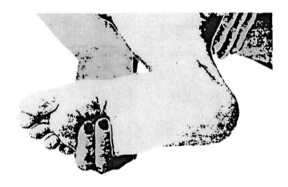

Exercise 4: Relieves Menopause-Related Insomnia

This exercise helps relieve insomnia and anxiety symptoms commonly experienced in menopause. In Chinese medicine, these points are called "joyful sleep" and "calm sleep".

Sit comfortably and hold these points for 1 to 3 minutes. Left hand holds point on the inside of the right anklebone. This point is located in the indentation directly below the inner ankle bone.

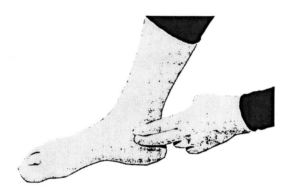

Right hand holds point located in the indentation below the right outer ankle bone. Repeat this exercise holding the points on the left foot.

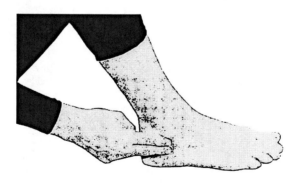

Exercise 5: Relieves Vaginal and Urinary Tract Atrophy and Promotes Healthy Bones

This exercise helps relieve symptoms of vaginal dryness and insufficient vaginal lubrication seen in menopausal women with inadequate estrogen stimulation of the vaginal tissues. These points are also used to promote strong and healthy bones. The second step in this sequence helps promote bladder health during menopause.

Sit on the floor with the knees bent or sit up and prop your back against a chair. Hold each step for 1 to 3 minutes.

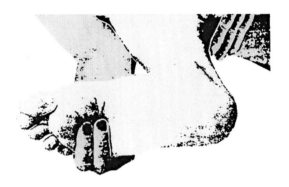

Right hand holds point at the base of the ball of the right foot. The point is located between the two pads of the foot.

Left hand holds the point midway between the inside of the right anklebone and the Achilles tendon. The Achilles tendon is located at the back of the ankle.

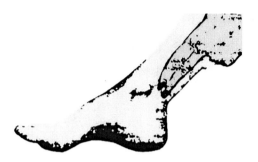

Move left hand 1 inch above the waist on the muscle to the side of the spine. Right hand holds the point on the outside of the foot, just behind the little toe.

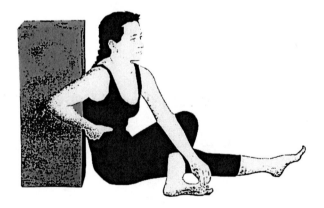

11

Cardiovascular Health

Exercise 1: Improves Cardiovascular Health

This exercise strengthens the cardiovascular system. Health problems involving this system are the major cause of death in postmenopausal women.

Sit or stand in a comfortable position. Hold each step for 1 to 3 minutes. Right hand holds point at the base of the armpit on the chest.

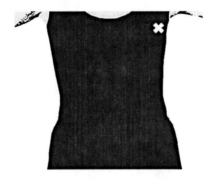

Right hand holds point at base of left wrist below the little finger.

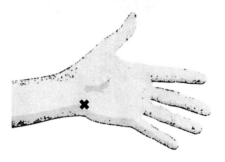

Exercise 2: Use for Relief of Anxiety Coexisting with Mitral Valve Proplase

This exercise helps relieve anxiety, nervous tension, and insomnia. It can also help relieve anxiety coexisting with mitral valve prolapse. It stimulates the entire endocrine system because it involves a powerful point for the pituitary gland. The points in this exercise also help relieve headaches, stiff neck, and stress-related breathing difficulties. This is also an effective exercise for relieving menopause-related hot flashes and hypoglycemia symptoms.

Sit upright on a chair. Hold each step for 1 to 3 minutes. Left hand holds spot located in the slight depression on the top of the head.

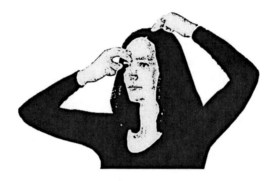

Right hand holds point directly between the eyebrows where the bridge of the nose meets the forehead.

Right hand holds point in the center of your breastbone, at the level of the heart. Your fingers will fit into the indentations in this bone.

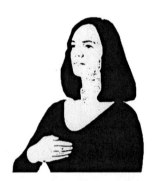

12

Breathing and Lung Health

Exercise 1: Use to Relieve Chest Tension

This exercise relieves anxiety causing chest tension and shallow breathing. It also involves a point that reduces hypoglycemia symptoms.

Sit comfortably. Hold each point 1 to 3 minutes. Left hand holds the point on the outer part of the chest. This point is located three finger widths below the collarbone.

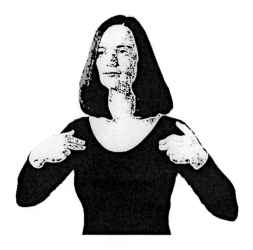

Right hand holds the same point on the right side.

Left hand holds a point on the right hand below the base of the thumb, in the wrist groove.

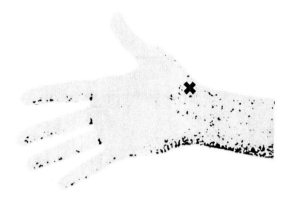

Left hand holds a point on the palm side of the right hand in the center of the pad below the thumb.

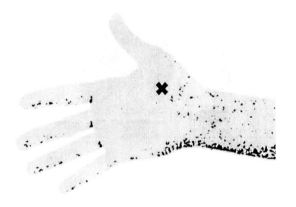

Exercise 2: Relieves Menstrual Stress and Fatigue, Breathing Difficulties due to Anxiety

This exercise helps relieve menstrual anxiety and depression, helpful to women suffering from significant stress in their lives. It helps relieve hot flashes related to the onset of menopause, as well as breathing difficulties caused by anxiety. The sequence of points relieves fatigue that many women experience for up to several days prior to the onset of their menstrual period. The second step in this sequence has traditionally been forbidden for use by pregnant women after their first trimester.

Sit up and prop your back against a chair or a wall. Hold each step 1 to 3 minutes. Right hand holds point at the base of the ball of the right foot. This point is located between the two pads of the foot.

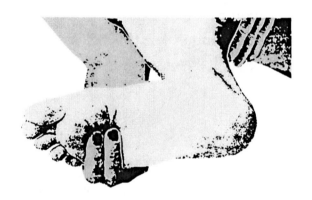

Left hand holds the point midway between the inside of the right anklebone and the Achilles tendon. The Achilles tendon is located at the back of the ankle.

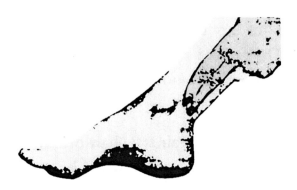

Left hand holds a point below right knee. Locate this point with right hand, measuring four finger widths below the kneecap toward the outside of the shinbone. It is sensitive to the in many people.

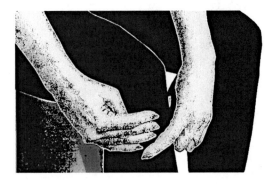

Exercise 3: Use for Relief of Breathing Difficulties and Anxiety Coexisting with Mitral Valve Proplase

This exercise helps relieve anxiety, nervous tension, and insomnia. It can help relieve anxiety coexisting with mitral valve prolapse. It stimulates the entire endocrine system because it involves a powerful point for the pituitary gland. The points in this exercise also help relieve headaches, stiff neck, and stress-related breathing difficulties. This is also an effective exercise for relieving menopause-related hot flashes and hypoglycemia symptoms.

Sit upright on a chair. Hold each step for 1 to 3 minutes. Left hand holds spot located in the slight depression on the top of the head.

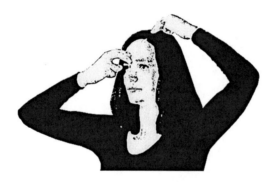

Right hand holds point directly between the eyebrows where the bridge of the nose meets the forehead.

Right hand holds point in the center of your breastbone, at the level of the heart. Your fingers will fit into the indentations in this bone.

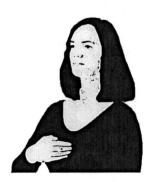

13

Breast Health

Exercise 1: Improves Breast Health

This point improves breast health by stimulating the pituitary, the master gland that regulates the output of hormones affecting the health of the breast tissue.

Sit upright in a chair or stand up. Hold each step for 1 to 3 minutes.

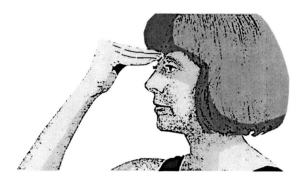

Right hand holds point directly between the eyebrows where the bridge of the nose meets the forehead.

Right hand holds point on right side of chest directly above the breasts in line with the nipples. Point is between the third and fourth ribs.

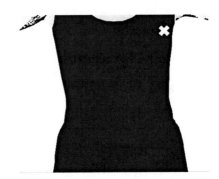

14

Thyroid Gland

Exercise 1: Use to Balance the Thyroid Gland

These points help normalize thyroid function and balance the thyroid gland. They also promote healthy skin tone and color.

Sit or lie in a comfortable position. Hold each step for 1 to 3 minutes. Left hand holds a point in the indentation behind the ear lobe.

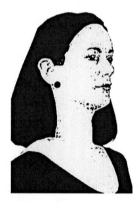 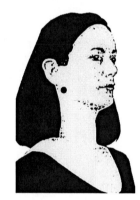

Then, left hand holds a point directly below the ear lobe and behind the jawbone.

Exercise 2: Use to Balance the Thyroid Gland

This exercise balances the thyroid gland. A hyperactive gland can cause anxiety and nervousness.

Sit upright on a chair. Hold each step for 1 to 3 minutes. Wrap hands around shoulders with thumbs pressing gently into both sides on top of collarbone.

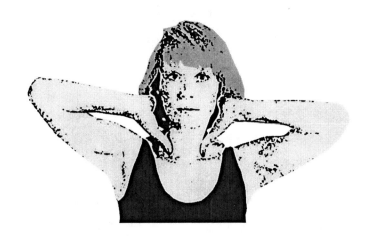

Fingers are in back. Press against upper shoulders and shoulder blade area.

Exercise 3: Relieves Thyroid Imbalance

This exercise energizes the thyroid, which can cause excessive menstrual bleeding.

Sit upright on a chair. Hold each step for 1 to 3 minutes. Wrap hands around shoulders with thumbs pressing gently into both sides on top of collarbone.

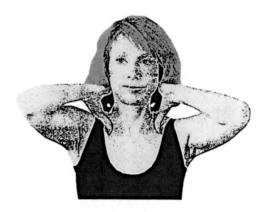

Fingers are in back and press against upper shoulders and shoulder blade area.

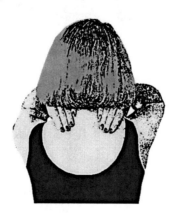

15

Digestive Health

Exercise 1: Use for Relief of Digestive Tension

This powerful energy point is one of the most important in Chinese medicine. It helps relieve digestive problems due to nervous tension and anxiety. It is also used to quickly diminish fatigue and improve energy and endurance. It has traditionally been used by athletes to tone and strengthen the muscles as well as increase stamina.

Sit upright on a chair. Hold the point for 1 to 3 minutes. Left hand holds a point below right knee.

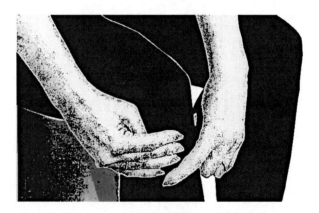

Locate this point with right hand, measuring four finger widths below the kneecap toward the outside of the shinbone. It is sensitive to the in many people.

Exercise 2: Use for Relief of Ulcer pain, Indigestion, Fatigue and Tiredness

This exercise helps relieve fatigue and tiredness. It stimulates the entire endocrine system because it involves a powerful point for the pituitary gland. This point also helps relax emotional tension as well as relieve eye strain, headaches, hay fever, ulcer pain, and indigestion.

Sit upright on a chair or against a wall. Right hand holds point directly between the eyebrows, where the bridge of the nose meets the forehead. Hold the point for 1 to 3 minutes.

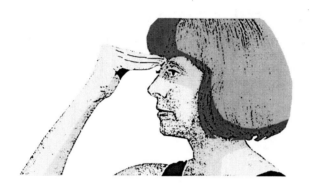

Exercise 3: Use for Relief of Hypoglycemia, Muscle Tension and Stress

This exercise includes a major treatment point for hypoglycemia. In addition, women who feel anxious and stressed often suffer from tight muscles. This important sequence of points helps relieve upper body tension. The neck and shoulders generally carry a great deal of tension. Tightness in this area can act as a bottleneck and impede the energy flow of the entire body. Thus, this sequence energizes the entire body, relieving fatigue and burnout as well as relieving anxiety and nervous tension. The points in this sequence also strengthen the immune system.

Hold each step 1 to 3 minutes. You will begin in a lying-down position and then sit upright on a chair. Fold a towel in half lengthwise. Lie down on your back and place the towel underneath your upper back between your shoulder blades, applying pressure to an important pressure point. Relax in this position for 1 to 3 minutes.

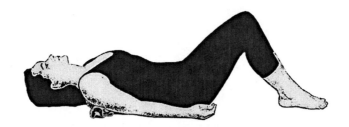

Now sit up. Left hand holds a point at the top of the shoulder blade, 1 to 2 inches to the side of the spine. The point is between the shoulder blade and the spine. It may feel firm and resistant.

Right hand holds the same point on the right side.

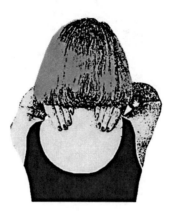

Left hand holds a point slightly to the back of the top of the shoulder where the neck meets the shoulder.

Right hand holds the same point on the right side.

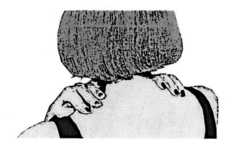

Left hand holds the point halfway on the neck; fingers rest on the muscle next to the spine.

Right hand holds the same point on the right side.

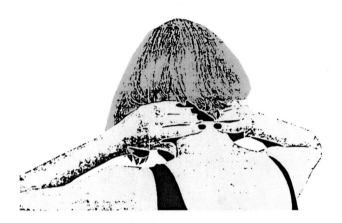

Left hand holds the point underneath the base of the skull, 1 to 2 inches out from the spine. Your fingers will feel a hollow spot at this point.

Right hand holds the point on the right side.

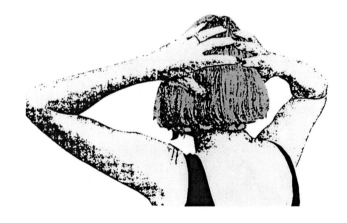

Exercise 4: Use for Relief of Hypoglycemia Symptoms

This is an effective exercise for relieving menopause-related hot flashes and hypoglycemia symptoms. This exercise also helps relieve anxiety, nervous tension, and insomnia. It can also help relieve anxiety coexisting with mitral valve prolapse. It stimulates the entire endocrine system because it involves a powerful point for the pituitary gland. The points in this exercise also help relieve headaches, stiff neck, and stress-related breathing difficulties. This is also an effective exercise for relieving menopause-related hot flashes and hypoglycemia symptoms.

Sit upright on a chair. Hold each step for 1 to 3 minutes. Left hand holds spot located in the slight depression on the top of the head.

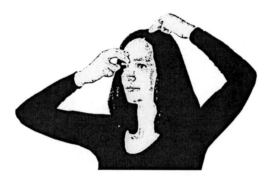

Right hand holds point directly between the eyebrows where the bridge of the nose meets the forehead.

Right hand holds point in the center of your breastbone, at the level of the heart. Your fingers will fit into the indentations in this bone.

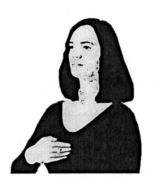

16

Headaches and Eye Strain

Exercise 1: General Balancing of the Energy Pathways and Relieves Headaches

This sequence of points balances the energy flow of the entire body and benefits all of the meridians. It is the most calming of all sequences because it works directly on the spine and the brain. It balances the entire nervous system. It is excellent in helping to relieve the anxiety, mood swings, and irritability that more than 80 percent of women with PMS seem to suffer. It relieves headaches and is also useful in balancing the energy of the reproductive tract.

Sit upright on a chair. Hold each step for 1 to 3 minutes. Left hand holds the point just below the base of the sternum. Right hand holds the point 2 inches below the navel.

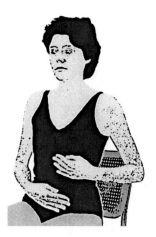

Left hand does not move. Right hand holds the point at the top of the pubic bone.

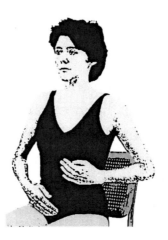

Left hand stays on the point just below the base of the sternum. Right hand holds the point at the bottom of the tailbone.

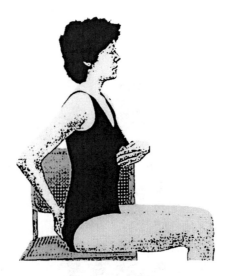

Left hand holds the point below the large vertebra (bone) at the base of the neck. Right hand is placed 1 inch above the waist on the spine.

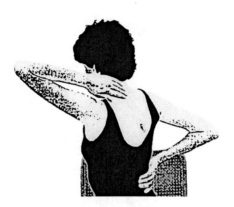

Left hand holds the point on the spine where it meets the base of the skull. Right hand stays 1 inch above the waist on the spine.

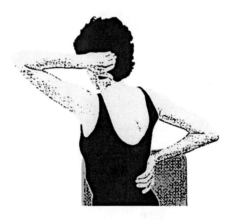

Left hand moves to the point between the eyebrows. Right hand holds the point on the top of the head.

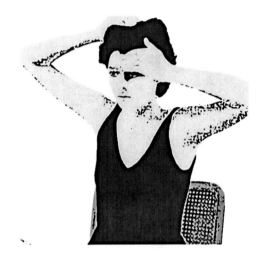

Left hand holds point between the nipples on the sternum.

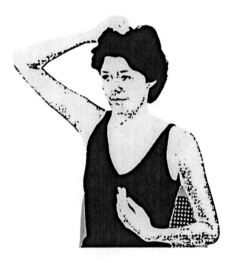

Right hand remains at the point on top of the head.

Exercise 2: Use for Relief of Headaches, Eyestrain, Fatigue and Tiredness

This exercise helps relieve fatigue and tiredness. It stimulates the entire endocrine system because it involves a powerful point for the pituitary gland. This point also helps relax emotional tension as well as relieve eye strain, headaches, hay fever, ulcer pain, and indigestion.

Sit upright on a chair. Right hand holds point directly between the eyebrows, where the bridge of the nose meets the forehead. Hold the point for 1 to 3 minutes.

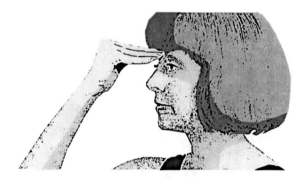

Exercise 3: Use for Relief of Headaches, Stiff Neck, Anxiety and Stress

This exercise helps relieve insomnia, anxiety, and nervous tension. It can also help relieve anxiety coexisting with mitral valve prolapse. It stimulates the entire endocrine system because it involves a powerful point for the pituitary gland. The points in this exercise also help relieve headaches, stiff neck, and stress-related breathing difficulties. This is also an effective exercise for relieving menopause-related hot flashes and hypoglycemia symptoms.

Sit upright on a chair. Hold each step for 1 to 3 minutes. Left hand holds spot located in the slight depression on the top of the head.

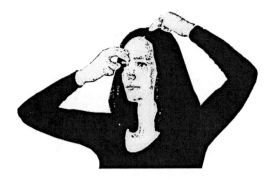

Right hand holds point directly between the eyebrows where the bridge of the nose meets the forehead.

Right hand holds point in the center of your breastbone, at the level of the heart. Your fingers will fit into the indentations in this bone.

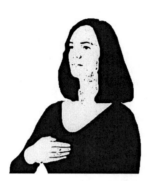

Exercise 4:Relieves PMS Related Headaches, Tightness of Neck and Shoulders, Depression and Hypoglycemia

The neck and shoulders generally carry a great deal of tension. Tightness in this area can act as a bottleneck and impede the energy flow of the entire body. Thus the entire body is energized by this exercise. It also relieves depression.

A major treatment point for hypoglycemia is worked on in this exercise. This may held reduce the excessive cravings for sweets that some women notice before their periods.

Sit comfortably or lie down. Hold each step 1 to 3 minutes. Left hand holds point at the top of the shoulder blade, 1 to 2 inches to the side of the spine. The point is between the shoulder blade and the spine. It may feel firm and resistant.

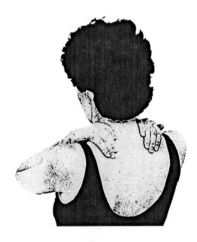

Right hand holds the same point on the right side.

Left hand holds points slightly to the back of the top of the shoulder where the neck meets the shoulder.

Right hand holds the same point on the right side.

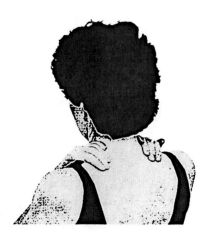

Left hand holds the point halfway up the neck; fingers sit on the muscle next to the spine.

Right hand holds the same point on the right side.

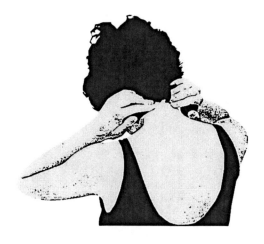

Left hand holds the point at the base of the skull 1 to 2 inches out from the spine.

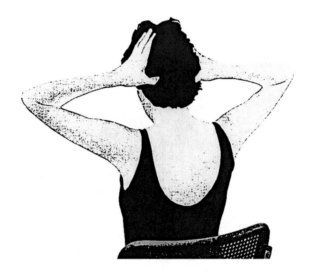

Right hand holds the same point on the right side.

17

Immune Function

Exercise 1: Improves Immune Function

This sequence of points strengthens the immune system and improves resistance to infections as well as relieving fatigue. This exercise also helps to prevent as well as relieve allergies. It balances the emotions and relieves symptoms of depression.

Sit comfortably or lie down. Hold each step for 1 to 3 minutes. Left hand holds point on right hand on the webbing between the index finger and thumb.

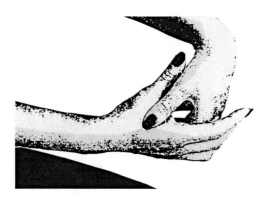

Left thumb is placed on top of the webbing and the index finger is placed underneath the palm. The webbing is squeezed between the thumb and index finger.

Left hand rubs firmly the area between the bones at the top of the left foot below where the big toe and second toe meet.

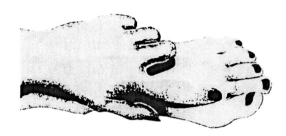

Left and right hands hold points one-half inch below the base of the skull. Fingers will press on the rope-like muscles on either side of the spine.

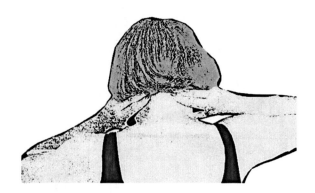

Left hand holds point two finger-widths below the navel.

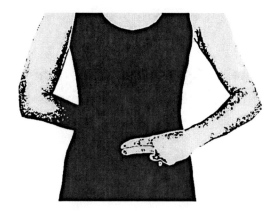

Left hand holds point below right knee. This point is located four finger-widths below the kneecap toward the outside of the shinbone. It is sensitive to the touch in many people.

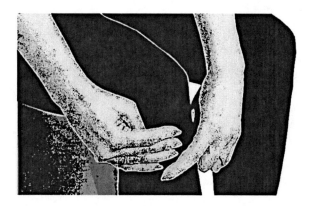

Exercise 2: Use for Relief of Hay Fever, Fatigue and Tiredness

This exercise helps relieve fatigue and tiredness. It stimulates the entire endocrine system because it involves a powerful point for the pituitary gland. This point also helps relax emotional tension as well as relieve eye strain, headaches, hay fever, ulcer pain, and indigestion.

Sit upright on a chair. Right hand holds point directly between the eyebrows, where the bridge of the nose meets the forehead. Hold the point for 1 to 3 minutes.

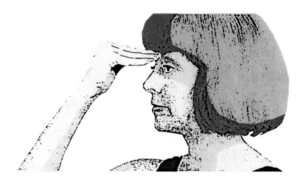

Exercise 3: Use for Relief of Fatigue, Depression, and Immune Dysfunction

This important sequence of points helps relieve upper body tension. The neck and shoulders generally carry a great deal of tension. Tightness in this area can act as a bottleneck and impede the energy flow of the entire body, thus releasing the tightness, energizing the entire body, and relieving fatigue. It also relieves depression and nervous tension. The points in this sequence also strengthen the immune system. A major treatment point for hypoglycemia is worked on in this exercise.

Sit comfortably or lie down. Hold each step for 1 to 3 minutes.

Left hand holds point at the top of the left shoulder blade, 1 to 2 inches to the side of the spine. The point is between the shoulder blade and the spine. It may feel firm and resistant.

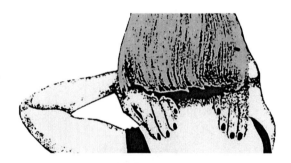

Right hand holds the same point on the right side.

Left hand holds point slightly to the back of the top of the left shoulder where the neck meets the left shoulder.

Right hand holds the same point on the right side.

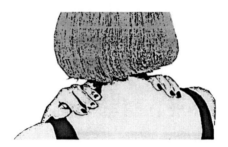

Left hand holds the point halfway up the left side of the neck. Fingers sit on the muscle next to the spine.

Right hand holds the same point on the right side.

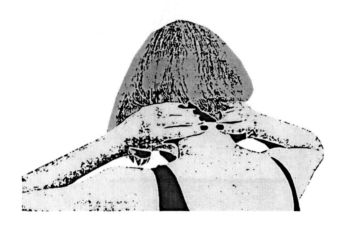

Left hand holds the point at the base of the skull, 1 to 2 inches out from the spine.

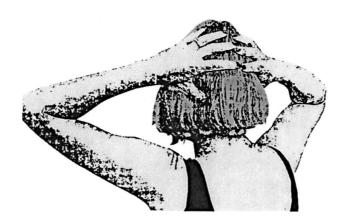

Right hand holds the same point on the right side.

Exercise 4: Use for Relief of Food Addiction

This exercise helps relieve food cravings and addictions for foods that worsen anxiety and nervous tension. Food addictions are often due to food allergies. This includes chocolate, sugar, and caffeine. This exercise also helps relieve anxiety and emotional stress, which often worsen digestive problems. Use this point on an empty stomach prior to eating. Do not hold this point deeply.

Sit or lie in a comfortable position. Hold this point for 1 to 3 minutes.

Right hand holds a point in the midline of the body, halfway between the bottom of the breast bone and the navel.

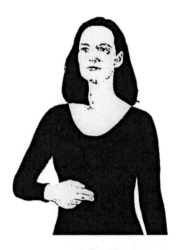

18

Insomnia

Exercise 1: Use for Relief of Anxiety and Stress

This exercise helps relieve insomnia, anxiety, and nervous tension. It can also relieve anxiety coexisting with mitral valve prolapse. It stimulates the entire endocrine system because it involves a powerful point for the pituitary gland. The points in this exercise also help relieve headaches, stiff neck, and stress-related breathing difficulties. This is also an effective exercise for relieving menopause-related hot flashes and hypoglycemia symptoms.

Sit upright on a chair. Hold each step for 1 to 3 minutes.

Left hand holds spot located in the slight depression on the top of the head. Right hand holds point directly between the eyebrows where the bridge of the nose meets the forehead.

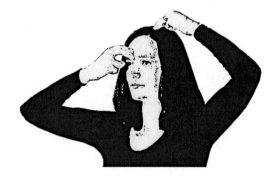

Right hand holds point in the center of your breastbone, at the level of the heart.

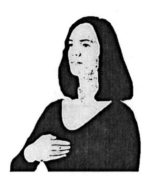

Your fingers will fit into the indentations in this bone.

Exercise 2: Use for Relief of Insomnia

This exercise helps relieve insomnia and anxiety. In Chinese medicine, these points are called "joyful sleep" and "calm sleep."

Sit comfortably and hold these points for 1 to 3 minutes.

Left hand holds the point on the inside of the right ankle. This point is located in the indentation directly below the inner ankle bone.

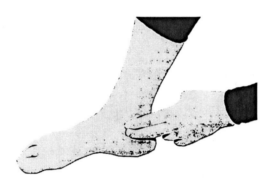

Right hand holds the point located in the indentation below the right outer ankle.

Repeat this exercise holding the points on the left foot.

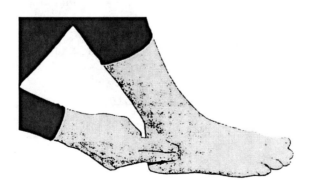

19

Anxiety and Stress

Exercise 1: Use for Relief of Anxiety and Stress

This exercise helps relieve anxiety, nervous tension, and insomnia. It can also help relieve anxiety coexisting with mitral valve prolapse. It stimulates the entire endocrine system because it involves a powerful point for the pituitary gland. The points in this exercise also help relieve headaches, stiff neck, and stress-related breathing difficulties. This is also an effective exercise for relieving menopause-related hot flashes and hypoglycemia symptoms.

Sit upright on a chair. Hold each step for 1 to 3 minutes.

Left hand holds spot located in the slight depression on the top of the head. Right hand holds point directly between the eyebrows where the bridge of the nose meets the forehead.

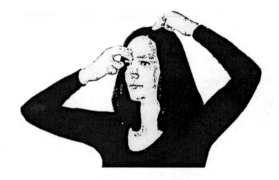

Right hand holds point in the center of your breastbone, at the level of the heart.

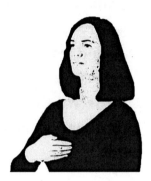

Your fingers will fit into the indentations in this bone.

Exercise 2: Use for Relief of Muscle Tension, Stress, and Hypoglycemia

Women who feel anxious and stressed often suffer from tight muscles. This important sequence of points helps relieve upper body tension. The neck and shoulders generally carry a great deal of tension. Tightness in this area can act as a bottleneck and impede the energy flow of the entire body. Thus, this sequence energizes the entire body, relieving fatigue and burnout as well as relieving anxiety and nervous tension. The points in this sequence strengthen the immune system and also include a major treatment point for hypoglycemia.

Hold each step 1 to 3 minutes. You will begin in a lying-down position and then sit upright on a chair.

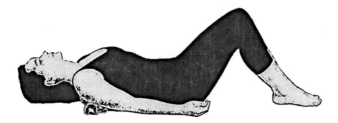

Fold a towel in half lengthwise. Lie down on your back and place the towel underneath your upper back between your shoulder blades, applying pressure to an important pressure point. Relax in this position for 1 to 3 minutes.

Now sit up. Left hand holds a point at the top of the shoulder blade, 1 to 2 inches to the side of the spine. The point is between the shoulder blade and the spine. It may feel firm and resistant.

Right hand holds the same point on the right side.

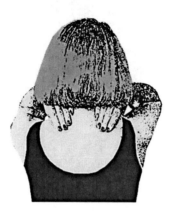

Left hand holds a point slightly to the back of the top of the shoulder where the neck meets the shoulder.

Right hand holds the same point on the right side.

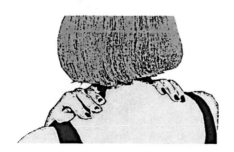

Left hand holds the point halfway on the neck; fingers rest on the muscle next to the spine.

Right hand holds the same point on the right side.

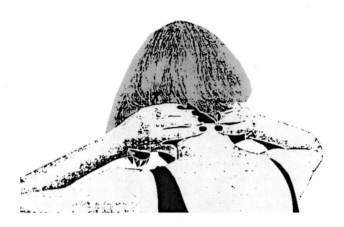

Left hand holds the point underneath the base of the skull, 1 to 2 inches out from the spine. Your fingers will feel a hollow spot at this point.

Right hand holds the point on the right side.

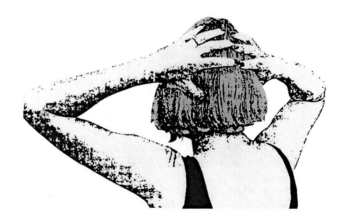

Exercise 3: Use for Relief of Insomnia and Anxiety

This exercise helps relieve insomnia and anxiety. In Chinese medicine, these points are called "joyful sleep" and "calm sleep."

Sit comfortably and hold these points for 1 to 3 minutes.

Left hand holds the point on the inside of the right ankle. This point is located in the indentation directly below the inner ankle bone.

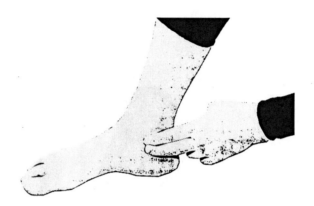

Right hand holds the point located in the indentation below the right outer ankle.

Repeat this exercise holding the points on the left foot.

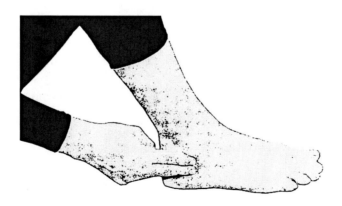

Exercise 4: Use to Relieve Chest Tension

This exercise relieves chest tension and shallow breathing caused by anxiety. It also involves a point that reduces hypoglycemia symptoms.

Sit comfortably. Hold each point 1 to 3 minutes.

Left hand holds the point on the outer part of the chest. This point is located three finger widths below the collarbone. Right hand holds the same point on the right side.

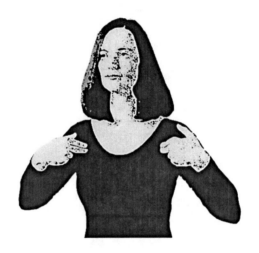

Left hand holds a point on the right hand below the base of the thumb, in the wrist groove.

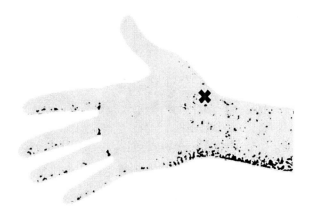

Left hand holds a point on the palm side of the right hand in the center of the pad below the thumb.

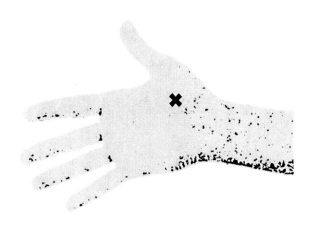

Exercise 5: Use for Relief of Digestive Tension

This powerful energy point is one of the most important in Chinese medicine. It helps relieve digestive problems due to nervous tension and anxiety. It is also used to quickly diminish fatigue and improve energy and endurance. It has traditionally been used by athletes to tone and strengthen the muscles as well as increase stamina.

Sit upright on a chair. Hold the point for 1 to 3 minutes

Left hand holds a point below right knee. Locate this point with right hand, measuring four finger widths below the kneecap toward the outside of the shinbone. It is sensitive to the in many people.

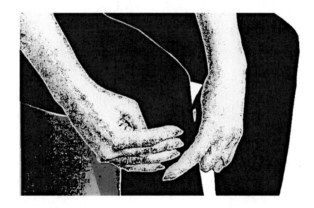

Exercise 6: Relieves PMS and Menstrual-Related Anxiety

This exercise relieves PMS symptoms and menstrual cramps by balancing points on the bladder meridian. This meridian relieves symptoms by balancing the energy of the female reproductive tract. Chinese medicine uses these points to relieve anxiety, fear, and exhaustion related to PMS, cramps, and other reproductive problems.

Sit on the floor and prop your back against a wall or a heavy piece of furniture. Hold each step for 1 to 3 minutes.

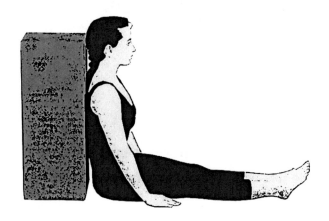

Alternative method: Lie on the floor and put your lower legs over the seat of a chair. Follow the exercise from that position.

Place left hand 1 inch above the waist on the muscle to the left side of the spine (muscle will feel firm and ropelike). Place right hand behind crease of the left knee.

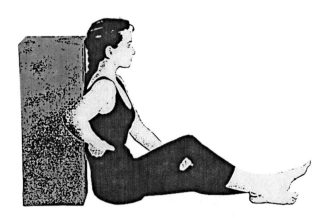

Left hand stays in the same position. Right hand is placed on the center of the back of the left calf. This is just below the fullest part of the calf.

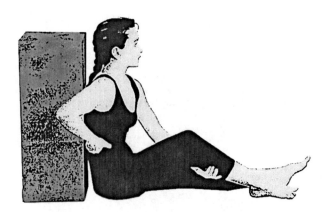

Left hand remains 1 inch above the waist on the muscle to the side of the spine. Right hand is placed just below the ankle bone on the outside of the left heel.

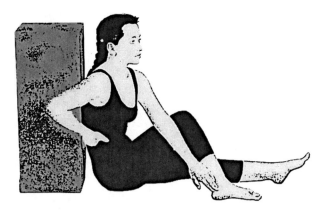

Left hand remains 1 inch above the waist on the muscle to the side of the spine. Right hand holds the front and back of the left little toe at the nail.

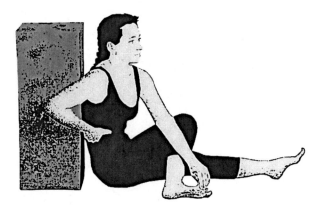

Exercise 7: Relieves Menstrual Stress and Fatigue

This exercise helps relieve menstrual anxiety and depression, helpful to women suffering from significant stress in their lives. It helps relieve hot flashes related to the onset of menopause, as well as breathing difficulties caused by anxiety. The sequence of points relieves fatigue that many women experience for up to several days prior to the onset of their menstrual period. The second step in this sequence has traditionally been forbidden for use by pregnant women after their first trimester.

Sit up and prop your back against a chair or a wall. Hold each step 1 to 3 minutes.

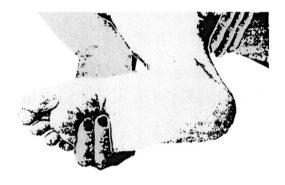

Right hand holds point at the base of the ball of the right foot. This point is located between the two pads of the foot.

Left hand holds the point midway between the inside of the right anklebone and the Achilles tendon. The Achilles tendon is located at the back of the ankle.

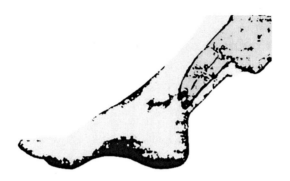

Left hand holds a point below right knee. Locate this point with right hand, measuring four finger widths below the kneecap toward the outside of the shinbone. It is sensitive to the in many people.

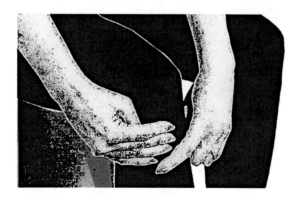

Exercise 8: Use to Balance the Thyroid Gland

These points help balance the thyroid gland and normalize thyroid function. A hyperactive glad can cause anxiety and nervousness. They also promote healthy skin tone and color.

Sit or lie in a comfortable position. Hold each step for 1 to 3 minutes.

Left hand holds a point in the indentation behind the ear lobe.

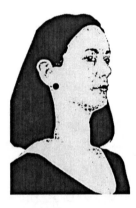 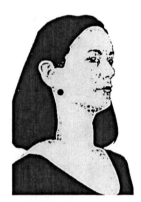

Left hand holds a point directly below the ear lobe and behind the jawbone.

Exercise 9: Use to Balance the Thyroid Gland

This exercise balances the thyroid gland. A hyperactive gland can cause anxiety and nervousness.

Sit upright on a chair. Hold each step for 1 to 3 minutes.

Wrap hands around shoulders with thumbs pressing gently into both sides on top of collarbone.

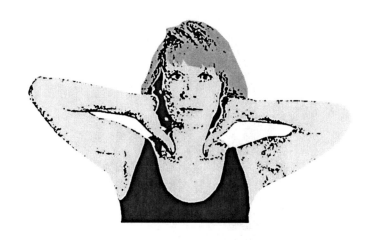

Fingers are in back. Press against upper shoulders and shoulder blade area.

Exercise 10: Use for Relief of Food Addiction

This exercise helps relieve food cravings and addictions for foods that worsen anxiety and nervous tension. This includes chocolate, sugar, and caffeine. This exercise also helps relieve anxiety and emotional stress, which often worsen digestive problems. Use this point on an empty stomach prior to eating. Do not hold this point deeply.

Sit or lie in a comfortable position. Hold this point for 1 to 3 minutes.

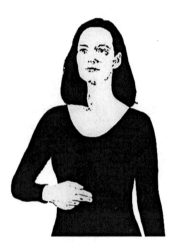

Right hand holds a point in the midline of the body, halfway between the bottom of the breast bone and the navel.

20

Tone and Strengthen Muscles and Increase Stamina

Exercise 1

This powerful energy point is one of the most important in Chinese medicine. It helps relieve digestive problems due to nervous tension and anxiety. It is also used to quickly diminish fatigue and improve energy and endurance. It has traditionally been used by athletes to strengthen and tone the muscles as well as increase stamina.

Sit upright on a chair. Hold the point for 1 to 3 minutes

Left hand holds a point below right knee. Locate this point with right hand, measuring four finger widths below the kneecap toward the outside of the shinbone. It is sensitive to the in many people.

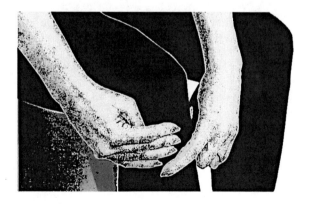

21

Chronic Fatigue and Tiredness

Exercise 1: Use for Relief of Fatigue and Tiredness

This exercise helps relieve fatigue and tiredness. It stimulates the entire endocrine system because it involves a powerful point for the pituitary gland. This point also helps relax emotional tension as well as relieve eye strain, headaches, hay fever, ulcer pain, and indigestion.

Sit upright on a chair. Right hand holds point directly between the eyebrows, where the bridge of the nose meets the forehead.

Hold the point for 1 to 3 minutes.

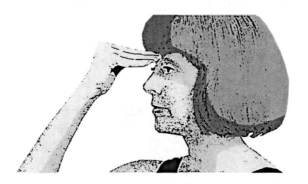

Exercise 2: Use for Relief of Fatigue, Depression, and Immune Dysfunction

This important sequence of points helps relieve upper body tension. The neck and shoulders generally carry a great deal of tension. Tightness in this area can act as a bottleneck and impede the energy flow of the entire body, thus releasing the tightness, energizing the entire body, and relieving fatigue. It also relieves depression and nervous tension. The points in this sequence also strengthen the immune system. A major treatment point for hypoglycemia is worked on in this exercise.

Sit comfortably or lie down. Hold each step for 1 to 3 minutes.

Left hand holds point at the top of the left shoulder blade, 1 to 2 inches to the side of the spine. The point is between the shoulder blade and the spine. It may feel firm and resistant.

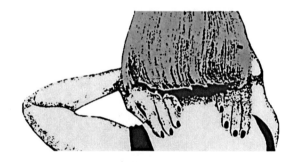

Right hand holds the same point on the right side.

Left hand holds point slightly to the back of the top of the left shoulder where the neck meets the left shoulder.

Right hand holds the same point on the right side.

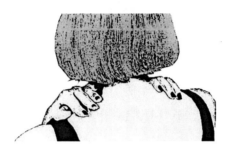

Left hand holds the point halfway up the left side of the neck. Fingers sit on the muscle next to the spine.

Right hand holds the same point on the right side.

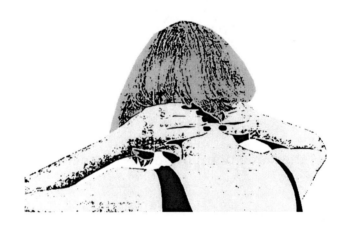

Left hand holds the point at the base of the skull, 1 to 2 inches out from the spine.

Right hand holds the same point on the right side.

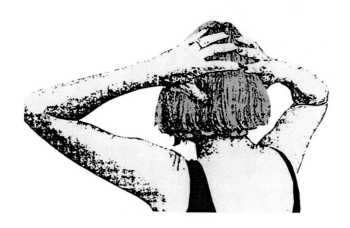

Exercise 3: Use for Relief of Fatigue and Tiredness

This exercise stimulates one of the most important acupressure points for energy, physical stamina, and power. The point stimulated in this exercise, termed the hara in Chinese medicine, is considered to be the body's center of gravity. This point also fortifies the digestive tract and helps to strengthen the reproductive system.

Stand or sit upright on a chair.

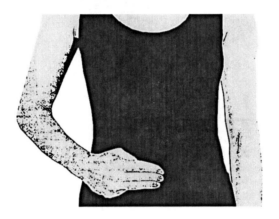

Fingers hold point below navel. Measure three finger-widths below navel to find this point. The point is located 1 to 2 inches deep inside the abdomen. Hold the point for 1 to 3 minutes.

Exercise 4: Use for Relief of Fatigue and Tiredness

This powerful energy point is one of the most important in Chinese medicine. It is used to quickly diminish fatigue and improve energy and endurance. Athletes have traditionally used it to tone and strengthen the muscles as well as increase stamina.

Sit upright on a chair.

Left hand holds point below right knee. This point is located four finger-widths below the kneecap toward the outside of the shinbone. It is sensitive to the touch in many people.

Hold the point for 1 to 3 minutes.

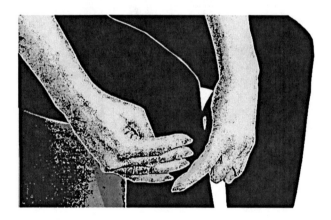

Exercise 5: Improves Immune Function

This sequence of points strengthens the immune system and improves resistance to infections as well as relieving fatigue. This exercise also helps to prevent as well as relieve allergies. It balances the emotions and relieves symptoms of depression.

Sit comfortably or lie down. Hold each step for 1 to 3 minutes.

Left hand holds point on right hand on the webbing between the index finger and thumb.

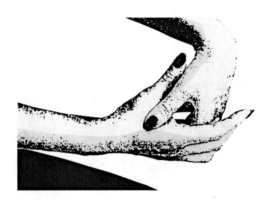

Left thumb is placed on top of the webbing and the index finger is placed underneath the palm. The webbing is squeezed between the thumb and index finger.

Left hand rubs firmly the area between the bones at the top of the left foot below where the big toe and second toe meet.

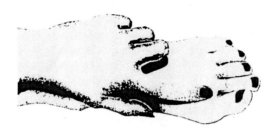

Left and right hands hold points one-half inch below the base of the skull. Fingers will press on the ropy muscles on either side of the spine.

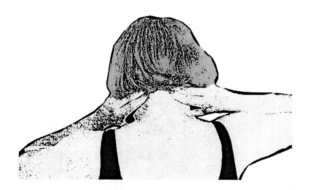

Left hand holds point two finger-widths below the navel.

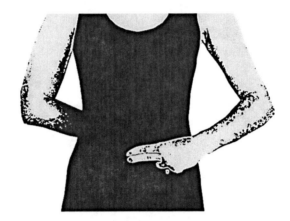

Left hand holds point below right knee. This point is located four finger-widths below the kneecap toward the outside of the shinbone. It is sensitive to the touch in many people.

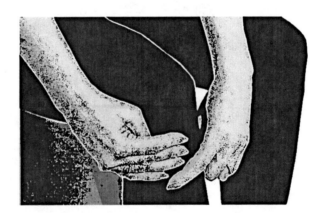

Exercise 6: Relieves Premenstrual and Menopausal Fatigue

This sequence of points relieves the fatigue that women experience prior to the onset of their menstrual periods. For many women with PMS, fati-gue is a significant problem that recurs every month. This exercise can also help to relieve menstrual anxiety and depression, as well as menopause-related fatigue. The second step in this sequence has traditionally been forbidden for use by pregnant women after their first trimester.

Sit up and prop your back against a chair. Hold each step 1 to 3 minutes.

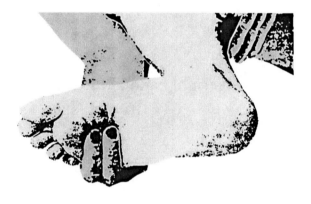

Right hand holds point at the base of the ball of the right foot. This point is located between the two pads of the foot.

Left hand holds the point midway between the inside of the right anklebone and the Achilles tendon. The Achilles tendon is located at the back of the ankle.

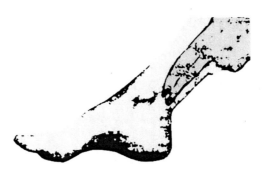

Left hand holds point on right hand at the base of fourth finger. Repeat sequence on left side.

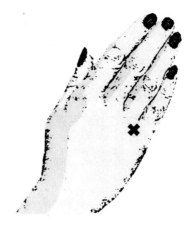

Exercise 7: Use for Relief of Thyroid Imbalance

This exercise energizes the thyroid, whose dysfunction can cause chronic fatigue and tiredness as well as excessive menstrual bleeding, anemia, constipation, and cold intolerance.

Sit upright on a chair. Hold each step for 1 to 3 minutes.

Wrap hands around shoulders with thumbs pressing gently into both sides on top of collarbone.

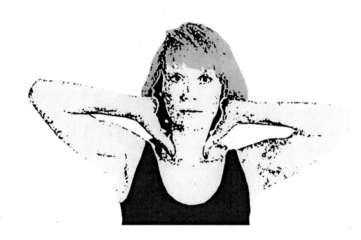

Fingers are in back. Press against upper shoulders and shoulder blade area.

Exercise 8: Use for Relief of Thyroid Imbalance

This exercise helps relieve chronic fatigue and tiredness due to thyroid imbalance. It is used to help stimulate the normal output of thyroid hormone.

Sit upright on a chair. Fingers touch three points along the large muscle on each side of the neck. Hold each point for 1 minute.

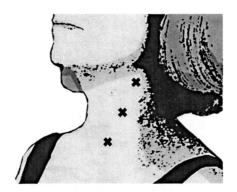

Exercise 9: Use for Relief of Anemia

This sequence of points is valuable for the treatment of anemia, a common cause of chronic fatigue and tiredness. This exercise involves stimulating points on the spleen meridian, related to blood formation and menstrual problems.

Sit upright on a chair. Hold each step for 1 to 3 minutes. Right hand holds a point four finger widths above the ankle bone.

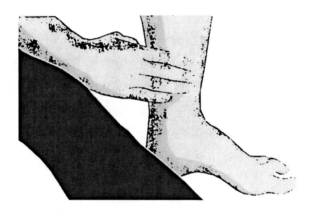

Left hand holds a point over the big toe.

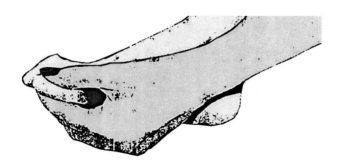

About Susan M. Lark, M.D.

Dr. Susan Lark is one of the foremost authorities in the fields of women's health care and alternative medicine. Dr. Lark has successfully treated many thousands of women emphasizing holistic health and complementary medicine in her clinical practice. Her mission is to provide women with unique, safe and effective alternative therapies to greatly enhance their health and well-being.

A graduate of Northwestern University Feinberg School of Medicine, she has served on the clinical faculty of Stanford University Medical School, and taught in their Division of Family and Community Medicine.

Dr. Lark is a distinguished clinician, author, lecturer and innovative product developer. Through her extensive clinical experience, she has been an innovator in the use of self-care treatments such as diet, nutrition, exercise and stress management techniques in the field of women's health, and has lectured extensively throughout the United States on topics in preventive medicine. She is the author of many best-selling books on women's health. Her signature line of nutritional supplements and skin care products are available through healthydirections.com.

One of the most widely referenced physicians on the Internet, Dr. Lark has appeared on numerous radio and television shows, and has been featured in magazines and newspapers including: Real Simple, Reader's Digest, McCall's, Better Homes & Gardens, New Woman, Mademoiselle, Harper's Bazaar, Redbook, Family Circle, Seventeen, Shape, Great Life, The New York Times, The Chicago Tribune, and The San Francisco Chronicle.

She has also served as a consultant to major corporations, including the Kellogg Company and Weider Nutrition International, and was spokesperson for The Gillette Company Women's Cancer Connection.

Dr. Lark can be contacted at (650) 561-9978 to make an appointment for a consultation.

We would enjoy hearing from you! Please share your success stories, requests for new topics and comments with us. Our team at Womens Wellness Publishing may be contacted at yourstory@wwpublishing.com. We invite you to visit our website for Dr. Lark's newest books at womenswellnesspublishing.com.

Dr. Susan's Solutions
Health Library For Women

The following books are available from Amazon.com, Amazon Kindle, iTunes, Womens Wellness Publishing and other major booksellers. Dr. Susan is frequently adding new books to her health library.

Women's Health Issues

Dr. Susan's Solutions: Heal Endometriosis

Dr. Susan's Solutions: Healthy Heart and Blood Pressure

Dr. Susan's Solutions: Healthy Menopause

Dr. Susan's Solutions: The Anemia Cure

Dr. Susan's Solutions: The Bladder Infection Cure

Dr. Susan's Solutions: The Candida-Yeast Infection Cure

Dr. Susan's Solutions: The Chronic Fatigue Cure

Dr. Susan's Solutions: The Cold and Flu Cure

Dr. Susan's Solutions: The Fibroid Tumor Cure

Dr. Susan's Solutions: The Irregular Menstruation Cure

Dr. Susan's Solutions: The Menstrual Cramp Cure

Dr. Susan's Solutions: The PMS Cure

Emotional and Spiritual Balance

Breathing Meditations for Healing, Peace and Joy

Dr. Susan's Solutions: The Anxiety and Stress Cure

Women's Hormones

DHEA: The Fountain of Youth Hormone

Healthy, Natural Estrogens for Menopause

Pregnenolone: Your #1 Sex Hormone

Progesterone: The Superstar of Hormone Balance

Testosterone: The Hormone for Strong Bones, Sex Drive and Healthy Menopause

Diet and Nutrition

Dr. Susan Lark's Healing Herbs for Women

Dr. Susan Lark's Complete Guide to Detoxification

Enzymes: The Missing Link to Health

Healthy Diet and Nutrition for Women: The Complete Guide

Renew Yourself Through Juice Fasting and Detoxification Diets

Energy Therapies and Anti-Aging

Acupressure for Women: Relieve Symptoms of Dozens of Health Issues
Through Pressure Points

Exercise and Flexibility

Stretching and Flexibility for Women

Stretching Programs for Women's Health Issues

About Womens Wellness Publishing

"Bringing Radiant Health and Wellness to Women"

Womens Wellness Publishing was founded to make a positive difference in the lives of women and their families. We are the premier publisher of print and eBooks focused on women's health and wellness. We are committed to publishing the finest quality and most comprehensive line of books that covers every area that a woman needs to create vibrant health and a joyful, fulfilling life.

Our books are written and created by the top health and wellness experts who share with you, our readers, their wisdom and extensive experience successfully treating many thousands of patients.

We encourage you to browse through our online bookstore; new books are frequently being adding at womenswellnesspublishing.com. Also visit our Lifestyle Center and Customer Bonus Center for more exciting and helpful health and wellness information and resources.

Follow us on Facebook for the latest health tips, recipes, and all natural solutions to many women's health issues (facebook.com/wwpublishing).

About Our Associate Program

We invite you to become part of the Womens Wellness Publishing Community through our Associate Program. You will have the opportunity to earn generous commissions on sales that you create through your blog, social network, support groups, community groups, school & alumni groups, friends, family or other networks. To join the Associate Program, go to our website and click "Become an Associate" (womenswellnesspublishing.com).

We support your sales and marketing efforts by offering you and your customers:

- Free support materials with updates on all of our new book releases, promotions, and bonuses for you and your customers
- Free audio downloads, booklets, and guides
- Special discounts and sales promotions

CPSIA information can be obtained at www.ICGtesting.com
Printed in the USA
LVOW09s1447271113

363064LV00018B/595/P

ML   9-14